Praise for P

"Jessie's experiences are ones we c...
women and femmes navigating so much to exist, thrive, and feel safe in these bodies. Jessie offers insight we can all use to find peace with ourselves. Like the rest of us, Jessie's path and inspiring insights haven't come without pain, challenge, devastation and the full spectrum of human emotion. We can all stand to listen to what others experience and share so vulnerably so we can learn compassion towards ourselves."

– Dana Falsetti, Yoga Instructor + Thought Leader @no-latrees

"Part confessional and part body acceptance roadmap, Project Body Love is a huge sigh of relief in a world filled with how-to's and 10-BEST-ways-to-figure-it-all-out. Author Jessie Harold bravely explores her experience in a way that feels both highly personal and highly universal. I caught myself nodding along, laughing, and crying with recognition as I read her words. This book is both a beacon of hope and a reminder that none of us are alone with our body confusion, fear, and shame, even when it might feel that way. Through Jessie's words, we have the chance to understand and feel the deep inner-working of the paradigm shift from diet mentality to a relationship with our bodies rooted in self-trust, purpose, and intuition."

- Mara Glatzel, MSW, intuitive guide and *Needy* podcast host

"Jessie's words feel like a homecoming. Having wrestled with the same weight issues and body love challenges all my life, I felt like this book offered a safe place to land in a world that doesn't always make our bodies feel welcome."

- Heather Plett, writer, coach, facilitator + teacher

"Our bodies are vulnerable. We get sick. We can't control their size. And, they will be the death of us. As a result, for most of us who have struggled with our bodies, they become a container for our vulnerability. In Project Body Love, Jessie clearly discerns what is her call to resilience, and our collective consciousness around not-thin bodies. Until we can separate the truth of our bodies from the truth of oppression, we will struggle to feel safe in our bodies. For those who want support around navigating the endless mystery the body is and offers, this book will help you come home to yourself."

-Ali Shapiro, MSOD, CHHC, *Insatiable* podcast host

"Harrold asks herself, 'What might have been possible if I hadn't spent so much time looking in the mirror? Reading about the next diet I would attempt?' Me too, Jessie, me too. What might be different about my life if I took all that energy + attention + wasted years I spent hating + fighting my body, and spent it elsewhere? What might our world look like if we all applied that energy elsewhere? I wish I had access to this book 20 years ago, but I take solace in the fact that this story will offer comfort to other women who are ready to be initiated into the power + wisdom of their bodies. Harrold uses her personal story of reclaiming her body, weaving in a fierce feminism and her academic background, to inspire us all to heal and to love these bodies of ours. Project Body Love is a fierce, honest, + necessary read for all women ready to transform their relationship with their body. Harrold's honesty moved me + her vision of healing inspired."

- Molly Mahar, Founder of Stratejoy

"A beautiful beacon of inspiration for anyone who finds themselves at a fork in the road and craves to finally return home to their temple, their body. Jessie decloaks her heart with refreshing honesty, as she guides her reader to an unconditional acceptance of self. Her heartfelt offering here is a genuine invitation to reunite with what matters most."

- Anne Berube, PhD, author of *Be Feel Think Do*

Project Body Love

my quest to love my body and the surprising truth I found instead

Jessie Harrold

Rebel Poet Press

DISCLAIMER: Project Body Love is the story of my own personal journey toward body acceptance, respect, and maybe even love. No part of this book contains medical advice, nor any formula for "success." Readers seeking their own version of body love should consult their intuition, physician or other trusted sources.

Cover photo by DeeDee Morris Photography. Cover illustration by Katika. Cover design by Joanna Price. Author photograph: DeeDee Morris.

ISBN: 978-1-9995444-0-9

First printing: December 2018

www.jessieharrold.com

Email Jessie Harrold at jessie@jessieharrold.com

"Don't write to get rich.
Don't write to get famous.

Write to get free."

— Desiree Adaway

"The skin can see…when you take a woman out of her skin and ask her to be something different than she really is, you literally blind her. You literally put out her eyes, her thousands of eyes that are all over the body."

— Clarissa Pinkola Estes, *The Joyous Body*

"Worldwide, the first and last steps to enslaving a woman are that she must be pleasing — that she must do as you say so, act as you say so, achieve an impossible norm that was not given to her as a gift at birth."

— Clarissa Pinkola Estes, *The Joyous Body*

For my body.

And for yours, too.

CONTENTS

Author's Note

I wrote this book not as an icon in the body positivity movement or as a fat activist with thousands of followers on Instagram and a flair for fashion.

I wrote this book as an ordinary woman who has, *like so many other women just like me*, spent the vast majority of my life hating and subsequently trying to change my body.

Well, I'm *almost* an ordinary woman who has always struggled with accepting, respecting, and loving my body. *Almost.*

I am also a teacher and life coach, and, in my work, I'm fiercely committed to supporting women to unearth themselves from beneath the expectations, roles, responsibilities and models of success - those externally-defined constructs of What Women Do – and reclaim who they are and what matters most to them – whether that's in their careers, their relationships, their parenting, their spirituality or, yes, in their bodies. After doing this work for a few years, I created a woman-centred model of change and a coaching methodology based on what I've learned about the complexity of disengaging from the personal and cultural narratives that challenge women's authenticity, sovereignty, and potential.

This book is an account of what happened when I used my methodology *on myself* in an attempt to disentangle from the impacts of society's expectations for my body, which I have spent a lifetime attempting and failing to live up to.

This book is, as all of my work is, both personal and political.

And I believe it's more imperative than ever: women are not just wasting their precious time, energy and money as they struggle to keep up to impossible body ideals. In both my life coaching work and my work as a doula (yeah, I do that too!), I have seen firsthand that, in so many ways, women's bodies are the seat of their personal power. They are the home of women's intuition and wisdom, the literal and metaphoric home within which the next generation will be nurtured, and, as posited by ecofeminists everywhere, a pathway to our society's renewed connection with the earth.

To me, the healing of women's relationship with their bodies is not just about the reconciliation of hundreds of years of commodification, hyper-sexualization, pathologization, shame and trauma. It is about reclaiming power and possibility, about restoring our culture's connection with the archetypal feminine, a deeply embodied power source that I believe can change the world.

But we start here. With this. With the thoughtful and compassionate dismantling of everything we've been told about our bodies, so that we can make way for what's possible.

We start here. With us.

Preface

This is the story of a quest – a Heroine's Journey, if you will – that I embarked on nearly three years ago. It's a story about my search for body acceptance, respect, and maybe even the elusive "body love."

But really, this is the story of a journey that began the first time my six-year-old self noticed the roundness of her belly, and tugged at the fabric of her Rainbow Bright t-shirt self-consciously.

And really, it's a story of a path that I'm *still* on.

This is my story, and so much of it is also the story of a million other women.

I decided to write this because salads weren't working anymore. Because going to the gym wasn't cutting it. Because I felt like there were deeper roots beneath my complex relationship with my body that longed to be unearthed.

I wrote this because I have wasted too much time trying to *change my body* into one that I felt like I could accept, respect, and love — a thinner body, to be exact. Because I knew that I was — and still am — a powerful, determined woman, and that if I were able to birth babies and businesses, climb mountains and swim oceans, but unable to successfully lose weight, then *something must be up. Something* must be wrong with this picture.

I wrote this because my inner feminist was so *totally* done with this. I've led an amazing life so far, and accomplished a great many things, but I can't help but wonder *what might have been possible* if I hadn't spent so much time looking in the mirror. Reading about the next diet I would attempt. Pining over the too-tight clothes in my closet.

I also can't help but wonder what might be possible for *society* if *the vast majority of women* weren't preoccupied with the skin-bound sack of flesh they were borrowing for this lifetime.

My first hope, when I sat down three years ago to begin this book, was to find healing for the fraught and often painful relationship *I've* had with my body. Writing has always been my catharsis, the way I make sense of myself and the world. My second hope was that by sharing my process and some of what I discovered both about myself and about the concept of body acceptance, respect and love in the context of our modern-day culture, that you may find some healing too. At the very least, you may find insight here. You may find a new perspective to consider.

I have always struggled with my weight, and I have, for the entirety of that always, been ashamed of that struggle. And so, despite the fact that I have often ruminated over meal plans and counted calories and steps and drops of sweat, I have rarely talked about my discomfort in my own body. I have, for many years, had a sort of emotional "no fly zone" about the issue, even in my own journaling. No Body Talk Allowed.

This book contains all the words I've never said. Because keeping it to myself hasn't worked, either.

INTRODUCTION

Why this? Why now?

After years of dieting and exercise propelled mostly by body hatred disguised as the pursuit of health and happiness, the question bears asking: why this? why now? What happened that made the rat race of weight loss finally so unacceptable that *this* was the time to finally end it?

I've spent an entire lifetime *wishing* I didn't feel so much loathing toward my body. Subsequently, I've spent an entire lifetime trying to starve or exercise those feelings away. And so a great part of this writing, this quest, was propelled by Albert Einstein's wise words:

"We cannot solve our problems with the same thinking we used when we created them."

But the other reason that I felt compelled to change my thinking toward my body was that the discomfort of being in my own skin began to take on an entirely new meaning when I ventured into entrepreneurship, and birthed my second child. My work as a life coach and wilderness quest leader held up a mirror, of sorts, to the way I was feeling about myself, and I couldn't ignore it, especially after my second pregnancy left me and my body riven with exhaustion and stretch marks.

And so, perhaps I'll start there - in the moments of despair and disorientation that catalyzed this whole personal quest to begin with.

Like so many women, I spent my 20s pursuing the goals that I believed were worthy based on my socialization within our culture: I had a burgeoning career with the public service, a beautiful home and one kid with another on the way.

But I didn't like my job and I felt horrible about how little time I spent with my child: I was working to make just enough money to pay for daycare fees so that someone else could look after her while I went to work. Which, in all honesty, wouldn't have been so bad if the work I was doing felt meaningful and impactful. But it didn't. I sat in my grey-walled cubicle all day, bored, and making plans for my escape.

My escape eventually took the form of entrepreneurship: I earned my life coaching certification, decided to ramp up my existing doula practice, and started a business. My husband and I decided to simplify our lives so that we could channel more of our personal resources into what mattered most, eventually downsizing to a small oceanfront bungalow and taking our kids out of full-time daycare. In short, I began to feel like I was more connected to who I *really* was and what mattered most to me; not completely unfettered but far less influenced by externally-validated models of success.

This urge to reconnect with oneself and one's values is a desire that I have found a great many of my peers and the women I coach with have been feeling. My theory is that there has been a confluence of events in recent years in our culture that has compelled us to question the ways in which we've been fitting into the boxes of "woman," "good mother," "sexy," "good partner," "successful." As I dove deeper into my own experience of this, and began to witness what the women around me were experiencing, I shifted my life coaching practice so I could help women learn to follow their internal compass for what feels true for *them* and what feels like living somebody else's life, with somebody else's goals.

And what happens when you find yourself in the business of seeking truth, of helping others step into greater authenticity?

I can tell you: you get Called to Attention.

All of a sudden, I found myself hyper-aware of the ways in which I was not living in integrity with my own values. I was cognizant of every time I did not speak my truth, every time I wore a facade of some kind. Though I had done so much of the work of shifting in my career and family life so that they better reflected who I was and what mattered to me, I felt a sense of misalignment in other aspects of my life that eventually couldn't be ignored.

Glaringly and consistently, I kept circling back to the increasing feelings of shame and animosity I was having about my body, which escalated after the birth of my second child.

8

My childbearing years had taken a toll on my physical shape, and my sense of acceptance hadn't caught up with that shape yet.

There was still a part of me that assumed I would shed that shape like a warm, maternal cloak, and I would return to the still-soft but much fitter, muscular and more able version of myself that I had come to identify with for so many years.

The other part of me was stymied by the fact that shedding this weight by the means I felt most familiar – eating "better" and exercising – was feeling extremely challenging as I learned to navigate the realities of having two children. I was tired. Like, really, really tired. Too tired for meal plans, or figuring out how to make grain-free oatmeal. Though I aspired to resume the amount of physical activity I was capable of in my pre-childbearing days, it was hard enough to take a poop by myself, let alone leave the house for an hour or more every day to attend to my physical health.

And so, eighteen months into my postpartum period with my second child, I felt like I was living in someone else's body – a body I couldn't recognize and did not want. I had gradually become physically unable to do many of the things I used to pride myself – even identify myself – as being able to do. I also felt bereft of the time and energy to pursue what I felt I needed to pursue to achieve better health.

These postpartum feelings certainly did their job intermingling with the desire to reconnect with myself and what mattered most to me – to my health and my ability and my sense of being at home in my own skin. I felt deeply compelled toward coming to peace with my body at long last.

And, admittedly, it wasn't lost on me that part of the reason I felt so negatively about my body was that the business I'd strived so diligently to create had me out in the public eye, leading retreats and workshops and women's circles on a regular basis. The social media presence required of me as a modern-day entrepreneur necessitated a great deal of public exposure. I believe that something happens to us when we see the lives of others on display in this way: we begin to subconsciously (or perhaps even consciously) place them on a pedestal. We make grand assumptions about people's lives based on what they present to the world as entrepreneurs, or as social media users. I began to get the sense that I was being perceived as someone who had her shit together – more than I felt like I did, anyway. I also began to get the sense that those who saw my "outsides," as portrayed to the public through my business and on Instagram and Facebook, were making assumptions about me and my validity as an entrepreneur based on the body they saw I inhabited when I posted pictures of myself.

How could someone who helps other people live in alignment with their values look like that? Doesn't that sense of alignment in one's life imply health? Doesn't thinness imply health?

Aren't all coaches and online entrepreneurs supposed to be blonde and bikini-clad and prancing in a sun-drenched meadow? (It's become an unfortunate part of what our society has come to expect that coaches do: here, look at my amazing life, and hire me to help you make your life as amazing as mine).

How could someone who leads wilderness quests in the backwoods be fat? How could I trust her with my life? She doesn't look like she could even climb a small hill let alone this mountain we're headed to...

There. I said it.

It was a dark and twisty space to occupy but I know that it's something that a lot of entrepreneurs and those in the public eye wrestle with, and it's not to be denied. I was not somehow so enlightened and autonomous and carefree that I had completely escaped the feeling of wondering if I lived up to others' expectations. Wondering what people thought of me. Wondering, in fact, if my body shape and its lack of congruence with what others see as healthy would affect my ability to succeed. Wondering if I deserved Success While Fat.

There. I said that, too.

And so, the confluence of my coaching work, my postpartum body angst, and the cognizance of my leadership and visibility in my community brought me to write this book. To search for a *new* way of thinking and being in my body, and to put an end to a lifetime of self-loathing, shame, and dieting. To find peace. Acceptance. Maybe even love.

THE BEGINNING

The *decision* to approach my relationship with my body in a new way, and to write about my process of doing so, was the simple part.

Next, I had to decide how I would actually *do it*.

Having spent the large majority of my life trying to lose some quantity of my physical mass, and generally proceeding henceforth into a cycle of joyful loss and equally exuberant re-gain, to say I was feeling extreme reluctance to dive into yet another diet or exercise regime or food diary-ing or mindful-ness practice as a part of this journey would be an enormous understatement.

None of those things had worked in the past, despite my deepest wishes to the contrary.

And a few years of life experience as well as the intensi-fied self-awareness that comes with being a life coach had me realizing that all those "solutions" I was slapping on the "problem" of the way my body looked were attempts to slap a *simple* solution on a *complex* problem.

It simply doesn't work. If it did, I would have "solved" this a long, long (long) time ago.

So would everyone else in our society who reports feeling uncomfortable in their skin, too fat, or unhealthy.

(even Oprah, I bet).

And so I decided to stop blaming myself for not having the will power, or shaming myself for not *wanting it badly enough*, or pointing fingers at media that I cannot change and cannot seem to "un-see." No. This time around I quickly realized that everything I had done up to this point to come around to feeling more like myself *in myself* was based on shitty logic.

This time around, I knew I needed to dive deeper into the complexity of my relationship with my body.

The Experiments

One of the practices that I encourage the women I coach with to do is to identify the area of their lives in which they feel least like themselves, least in integrity with who they are and what matters most to them, and then to design a series of tiny experiments to see if they can start to shift that experience.

This method is called safe-to-fail experimentation, and it's rooted in a paradigm called complex adaptive systems theory – the idea that there are "simple problems" that can and should be solved with "simple" solutions, and then are "complex problems" that require a much more nuanced approach. The idea behind safe-to-fail experimentation is that you try to learn more about the "problem" you're trying to solve by designing shifts — tiny experiments — that might impact the situation, and then observing what happens. *Learning* is the key here: the assumption in this practice is that if you already knew the solution, or even the nature of the problem, you wouldn't *have* a problem any more. If that were the case, dieting would have worked for me (*and Oprah*) a long time ago. Keeping the experiments small and incremental also makes them "safe-to-fail" and very doable — there are no grand gestures or elaborate plans that feel impossible to begin and daunting to implement. Just small nudges in what *might* be the right direction, followed by efforts to magnify what works, and stop doing what doesn't work.

Aha.

And so, after much hemming and hawing and soul-searching about what to do with the feelings I was feeling, I realized I needed to take a dose of my own medicine. I needed to create a series of tiny experiments that I believed might get me closer to feeling the way I wanted to feel *about* my body and *in* my body.

A list of experiments came to me over the course of a few weeks of simply setting the intention to discover what might make me feel more at home in my body. Some of the experiments came from the lens of self-care, some from the perspective of self-acceptance and self-love, and others from the perspective of my health and physical ability, and how those aligned with the life I desired for myself.

With no promises to myself as to outcomes or time-lines, I just dove in. I started with the experiments that felt the easiest, most urgent or most fun, and allowed the more complex shifts to continue to percolate in the meantime.

The remainder of this book is a chronology of that experimentation.

And, in fact, writing this book has been a part of the experimentation, in and of itself.

(meta, I know)

Because writing this book was, if nothing else, a great decloaking from a layer of shame I've held for the entirety of my adult life. Shame about even *feeling* the way I felt about my physical body. I always felt as though, as an intellectual woman with bigger fish to fry in *every* other area of her life, that dwelling on my shape was playing really small in the Big Game. I deeply wanted to be a woman who was confident and at peace with herself. I didn't *want* to have so much of my energy consumed by unhelpful thoughts about the way my fat felt on my butt or what I ate for dessert or why I couldn't stop myself from binging and just go for a run. All this felt incredibly silly and unimportant.

And yet.

And yet it truly did consume a frightening amount of my headspace.

I wondered, often, how much more I would have been capable of if I didn't have all those stories of my personal worth vis-à-vis my physical body pacing around my grey matter day in and day out.

Literally, all. day. long.

So there. I said it, anyway.

The way I looked, physically, was something that caused me years pain and shame and deep self-loathing.

I didn't want to feel that way anymore. Ironically, regardless of how I looked.

PART ONE

Tiny Experiments: Year One

— awakening —

The History Experiment

My first experiment was a thorough investigation of the history of my body, and my relationship with it. It was a way of orienting myself to the shift I was trying to make in my thinking about my body: my hope was that by doing this, I might excavate some long-held beliefs, family stories, and patterns that would give me some insight, some clues about how I might begin to create a new way of thinking about myself.

Letitia and the Fat Witch

The first photo of myself in which I recognized physical "imperfection" was one that was taken when I was just about five years old.

Five.

I was standing in the driveway of my childhood home, wearing, as many of us did in the 80s, extremely short terrycloth shorts, white socks up to my knees, a Rainbow Bright tee shirt, a red sun visor and some extremely large red sunglasses. In this photo I stand there, grinning at the camera, my belly protruding, my shorts pulled up over my little-kid paunch.

I was a fat kid.

I recall this fact as being quickly and audibly vocalized by the people that surrounded me.

"She looks just like Letitia," my aunt would say.

I had no idea who Letitia was, but I knew that the subtext of this comment was that Letitia was *fat*.

My next memory of my fatness was when I visited an interactive discovery centre as a kid. There was an activity there that I interpreted to be about choosing *all* the foods that were healthy from a selection of photos, and then entering these into a computer to be scored. Evidently I got the purpose of the activity wrong: I was supposed to just enter the foods that would make *one* healthy meal. The computer printout came out and it read, in no fewer words, that I was a pig. This *was* the 80s, but still.

I was a witch for Halloween a few years earlier, or later — the timing, I suppose, doesn't matter as much as the permanency of the memory. When I arrived at the doorstep of a neighbourhood woman, she responded to herself after asking, "well what have we here" with "oh! a fat witch."

I still remember, perhaps many years later, although I can't say for sure, a close family member telling me my arms looked like slabs of meat. Or steaks, or something. It was the only directly derogatory comment I remember coming from a loved one, and for the most part, my memory of others' perceptions of my fatness as a child was more in the form of sidelong glances and cryptic statements than outright shaming or even attempts to control my weight. But I still, sometimes, look in the mirror and before I know I'm even doing it, I say to myself "those arms look like slabs of meat."

It didn't help that I was a fairly quiet kid who much, much preferred sedentary activities to more active ones. I spent my Grade Five recesses not playing dodgeball, but writing a novel, huddled up against the prairie winter wind in a nook along the side wall of the school. I would pretend I was sick on track and field days, because of the burning feeling in my chest when I ran an entire loop of the track, and because I didn't want one of the Bronze medals that all the fat kids got.

Interestingly, looking back upon the photos from those days, I'm not sure if I ever was truly fat — definitely not among my leaner peers, but, looking back, I wonder if I simply began to live into the perception that others had of me, the label that they used to describe me.

Eating Like a Bird

I come from a family of women who Eat Like Birds. They are the sort, like so many of their generation, who "couldn't possibly eat another bite," will "just have a sliver," and "don't need anything." They even go so far as to identify themselves to others on a regular basis as *people who rarely eat very much*. They do not need to be worried about when someone else is cooking for them or offering them nourishment.

But me? I will always have another bite, a hefty piece, and I will always need when I need, want when I want. I will eat my kid's pie, if it means I can have pie. No martyrdom here, not even in the name of love, and definitely not in the name of smallness.

Nevertheless, this family story quickly taught me the shame of overeating, or indulging in too many sweets, and so I did these things in private. I would hide behind cupboard doors or just hope that no one would notice when I stealthfully reached for seconds and thirds. I could not eat like a bird, and so I hid instead.

Reinvention and Shame

My first Reinvention – that I can remember, anyways – was when I was in Grade Five. That was the year that I remember beginning to notice myself as being larger than the other kids in my class. That was also the year, I distinctly remember, that I reached the milestone weight of 100 pounds.

I don't remember ever having weighed myself before that point, and I don't remember what motivated me to do so at the tender age of ten, but there it was. One hundred pounds. The only thing I can recall is that my judgement of that number included the belief that it was *more than the rest of my friends*.

This would be a recurring theme for me — this comparison of myself to my friends. I believe that my first experiences of comparison were not necessarily the fuel for derisive self-talk in the way I find they became later on in my life, but they did prove to reinforce that I was *different* in some way than my friends were. There was a whole raft of experiences that I had as a 100 pound child — agonizing over wardrobe choices that looked acceptable, feeling the roll of my belly escape from the elastic top of my pyjama pants — that I assumed no other 10 year old child, at least in my small circle of friends, had. In fact, this experience of my body's size remained well into my adulthood: it was often not one of negative self-perception so much as it was one of alone-ness.

These feelings fuelled a desire to reinvent myself, and I did so with regularity. My efforts now seem somewhat laughable in their ineffectiveness, but I was earnest in my attempts. During breaks away from my friends — Spring Break and especially summer break — my goal became to return to my circle of peers *utterly unrecognizable* as compared to the fat girl they had once known. I can't recall these attempts including anything as pragmatic as dieting or exercising until my teen years; in those early days, my focus was primarily on fashion and hairstyles.

On this particular reinvention effort — that first one I remember in Grade Five — I located an old shirt of my father's and some jeans I no longer wore, and used that puffy neon bake-in-the-oven fabric paint to decorate the clothes with flowers and other designs. With my dad's help, I sewed myself a matching hair scrunchie, and with that, I was prepared to meet my peers once more. Different. Changed. Not who they thought I was.

Nothing changed, really, when I showed up to school in my brand new, self-styled outfit, except perhaps that I satiated my need to have some control over the way I presented myself to the world, and, hopefully, to the way I was perceived by others. Briefly, I believed that neon fabric paint might ease the pain of not-belonging that my fatness made me feel.

The compulsion to become someone different than I was began to narrow in its focus and became about my weight — what I now understand was my primary dissatisfaction with myself — in my teen years. Assuming exercise was the key to my success, I summoned the immense courage to appear *running in public* in the very small town in which I grew up. This, to me, was potentially very shameful, and I worried that others would see me running. I suppose, at the time, the town I lived in was not one in which people were regularly seen out running (the culture of my hometown was to enjoy other kinds of outdoor activities suited to the natural environment, like skiing or swimming, and hence, not activities that could be seen as being done solely for the purpose of *exercise,* as I assumed running to be). Being seen running, particularly being a fat girl seen running, could only mean one thing: that I was trying to lose weight. And to be seen doing that would be to be seen admitting that I was fat and needed changing.

Years later, in writing about this experience, I realized that I have been, and was, so shameful of my weight that it was even shameful to admit that I wore it on my body, and that I was dissatisfied with it.

That had been a primary experience of mine, in fact: that I felt ashamed to even admit I was ashamed with my body, and that I recognized it as fat, and that I recognized fat as something I didn't want to be. This, like a denial of my own self-denial. It is why negative self-talk and the compulsion to diet weren't as natural an extension of my challenges accepting my body as they were for others – I had a hard time even allowing myself to think: I AM fat. This was something that changed over the years, and I gradually became more willing to admit my shame to others, if only because I felt "supported" by a greater awareness, thanks to social media, of others who felt the same way. At the time, though, fat was not only something I didn't want to be; I was deeply ashamed even to admit that I waged an ongoing internal battle with my weight.

Reinvention continued to be a theme for me throughout my life, and thanks to goodness-knows-what social influences and personal thought processes, it always carried with it an assumption that I would not only emerge from my reinvention thinner, but that being thinner would also mean that I would be happier, and that I would be able to choose clothes from my wardrobe quickly and easily (*this desire has always been with me; an assumption that thin people skip that step in the beginning of their day that involves standing in front of a mirror, picking at the places their clothes cling too tightly, and then deciding to wear something completely different*). I assumed that my weight loss, my transformation, would find me not just thinner but more energetic. Not just attractive but *glowing.*

Oh, to glow.

The reinventions continued, even until very recently, and, being older and wiser, those *other* reasons to lose weight — to be happy, to be able to keep up with my kids, to *glow* — were what I would happily claim were my motivations for *being seen* exercising or limiting my food intake (which have, I suppose, become a bit more de rigeur in our society now, and for a grown woman, in a way they weren't when I was a teen and all my friends weighed ninety pounds soaking wet).

But there remained, especially in my later years, a deep-rooted shame in admitting that I might want to lose weight *just to look good.*

To look *normal,* I think, is how I had always felt. To have what I long believed to be a *normal* experience of my body, not fraught with all the inconveniences and shamefulnesses of fat.

All this served to separate me and my experience of my body from others. Though in my adult years I found friends who experienced similar dissonance in their bodies — *even (even!)* women who were actually not, technically, fat (!!) — I still held the idea that *this is not normal. I am not normal.* Thin is normal, and the thin experience is one I desire. Looking back on the reinvention processes I would put myself through, I now see one thing starkly that I didn't then: they involved me isolating myself from my friends and family so that I would return into the fold dramatically different. I craved their startled, surprised and pleased reactions when I would (fictionally, because I never truly did *actually* reinvent myself very successfully) return from my cocoon of my personal (and mostly physical) transformation. And so as a result, I did the one thing I probably shouldn't have: I made the feelings I had about my body my own alone, isolated myself, assumed no one was having similar experiences, and shamed myself for even feeling that way.

It occurs to me now that when I grew into a young adult and acquired a passport and some disposable income, the handful of gap years I took during university were not so much about taking a break and finding myself but LOSING MYSELF so as to return as someone more acceptable, somehow. Someone more worldly, with more life experience, and, hopefully, someone with a tan and about thirty less pounds to her name.

I don't have this same desire to transform myself now; not really. I have become more comfortable with many aspects of myself, if not my body. I have fewer delusions that becoming thinner will change very much other than my mass. Fewer. Not none, but fewer. *(The allure of glowing still remains, despite the fact that I now see this as a vestige of the diet industry. What is it about positively "glowing" that can sell a woman a diet? I'm not sure, but I've been sold for years.)*

False Acceptance

Alongside my lifelong attempts at reinventing myself, I had often, in my life, found myself in situations where I had to face my feelings about my physical appearance and *do something with them, quick-fast*, in order to survive. These experiences also prominently mark the history of my relationship with my body.

One of these situations was during my years of lifeguarding, from the tender age of sixteen until I was twenty-five.

My first few years lifeguarding — as I was achieving the final certificates of my training — I was not a fast or fit swimmer, by far. But after I moved away from my small town and applied for more competitive jobs in the city where I went to university, I realized I had to up the ante when it came to my lifeguarding fitness.

This ended up being the beginning of a fitness obsession that continued throughout my twenties. Although my motivations for physical fitness changed as the years went on, my original inspiration for improving my swimming and my cardiovascular health wasn't laden with the feelings I had about my body so much as it was rooted in the desire to actually be able to save someone who was drowning in the pool where I worked, if it ever came down to it.

Lifeguarding wasn't just about swimming fast and saving people, though. Anyone who's watched *Baywatch* knows that lifeguarding also requires a person to spend a great deal of time in one's bathing suit. During the time that I spent watching over the pool, I had to come to what I see now as a sort of false acceptance of my body. It was a given that we, as lifeguards, were to wear a bathing suit, maybe a mesh tank top over top of that (with the hem tucked in the upper thigh seams of the bathing suit, as was cool at the time)…and not much else. I felt uncomfortable being so scantily clad in public. And it wasn't just that — it was that I had to use my scantily-clad body in a very functional way; I could not hide or pose myself; I had a job to do that required me, in short, *to just get on with it.* To sit and squat and run and carry massive jugs of chlorine. I couldn't afford to think too carefully about how I looked or how I might be perceived by other pool patrons.

And so I managed to ignore the feelings of discomfort I had in my own skin. Quite effectively, in fact. It felt like acceptance, but I knew it was false.

I came to notice that the same thing would happen when I was to become intimate with someone new in some way: I would just *get over* my body insecurity. It was like my brain was capable of just short-circuiting the stories I had about whether my body was too big, or what the person who was to see me with fewer clothes on would think. Perhaps it was a survival mechanism, but it was *lovely*. For just that moment, I would be free from the negativity I felt about how I looked, simply because, it the truest sense of the phrase, *it was not serving me anymore.*

It makes me wonder, though: how on *earth* was it serving me the rest of the time?

The Fit Years

After having spent my formative years fairly sheltered from the notion of diet and exercise as a means of transforming my body, in my twenties, the world of diet culture and the thin ideal increasingly became my reality. It started slowly and fairly innocently, as I began to identify new ways of relating to my body and to physical activity.

Something happened to *me* when my dad went through what our family jokingly refers to as his mid-life crisis. My family was never an *inactive* family, I wouldn't say: like many of the families in the town where I grew up (which was an unusual place in that there were so many incredible outdoor activities to partake in: swimming, golf, cross country skiing, biking and more — we were outside most of the time that the weather warranted). I recall a modicum of "screen time": mostly *Saved by The Bell* on weekends, in my formative years. Our lives were oriented toward physical activity, but we weren't fanatical about it; it was just something we did. About the time when my dad turned forty-five, he, propelled by the early chronic disease and deaths of his parents, starting taking on more vigorous, intentional and sometimes grandiose physical endeavours. In those first years, he took up rowing, and he also participated in the local triathlon, an event held every year that drew participants from all over Canada.

I distinctly remember thinking, at the time, that I would *not* be outdone by my father. I had the sense that he was rapidly becoming more physically fit, at nearly fifty, than I was as I neared the end of my teenage years. This disturbed me to no end, and I started to consider physical activity as more than something I did with my family to pass the time. I started to see exercise through the lens of health, by the example that my dad set.

Something else happened around this time, too: I had a pivotal experience after a close call with a hulking wall of white water that made me realize that not only was a physically fit body my ticket to better health (and, mostly, outdoing my dad) but that *my body could do cool things.* Things that made me pretty darn cool, myself.

On a routine visit to my maternal grandparents' house when I was sixteen, my dad and I decided to go whitewater rafting. This was not something we'd ever discussed doing before, and I don't remember what possessed us to attempt this daredevillish feat. I was a great swimmer at this point, but I had never done anything to challenge my body or my derring-do in this way.

On our whitewater adventure, we had a fun time with lots of laughs and a bit of hard paddling, all up until the final rapid of the day. It was a "5+" meaning, in whitewater language, really fucking big. We were all briefed on how we would help navigate the boat, avoiding a massive standing wave that would effectively crush us on the left of the river, as well as a gigantic whirlpool that would suck us into oblivion (my interpretation only) on the right hand side of the river. We were to paddle when the guide said "paddle," and listen carefully to all instructions.

You know where this is going. The boat flipped, very early on into the run, and the entire contents of the boat (meaning, myself, my dad, and some eight other poor souls) ended up swimming down the heaving beast of a river. I thought I would die, I thought my dad would die, I totally *did* get sucked into the Whirlpool of Oblivion and at the end, I pulled myself up onto a rock, found my dad had made it down, too, with great relief, *and was utterly transformed.*

I can almost still feel the endorphin and adrenaline cocktail that must have been surging through my body after our harrowing whitewater experience. The message that my body got was: you can do hard things, doing hard things is actually kind of fun, and, it feels really fucking good to do hard things. Also: doing hard things is cool. It felt like a recipe for acceptance after spending my childhood in a body that never quite belonged.

As that year of my late-teenage life progressed, resplendent with possibility and extra confidence, I decided I would train for and participate in the local triathlon. For the first time I didn't feel that I would be under the scrutiny of the nosier folks in my small community: a fat girl trying to get thin (and thereby admitting that she was fat). No: I was running and biking and swimming because I was a fat girl about to participate in my first race.

I was beginning to develop a schema of myself as someone who was Physically Capable of Things. The pride I felt at being able to Do Cool Things almost — *almost* — usurped the horrible feelings I had about my physical appearance. Perhaps there was a slight bit of rebelliousness in it all: you don't think my fat body can Do Cool Things? Just watch.

I signed up for high school varsity soccer; I learned to shoot a gun and ran a biathlon. I went on my school's annual bike and canoe trips — multi-day excursions that were the *absolute* highlight of every kid's year in our school. I signed up for the varsity golf team, even though we mostly just rented golf carts and spun doughnuts on the edges of the fairway when no one was looking. I spent hours and hours rollerblading around the smooth roads of my hometown with my best friends. All this still didn't feel like *exercise,* per se: just a way to spend the time in a small town where there was little else for a teenager to do.

When I left home, in my first and second year of university, being physically active wasn't exactly my main priority. There was unlimited chocolate milk in the cafeteria and friends to be made. Living in my very first apartment, I spent a lot of my time watching Survivor and trying to figure out how to cook meals myself and my two roommates could enjoy, which usually resulted in eating peanut butter, chocolate chips and mini rainbow marshmallows in *utterly perfect* proportions squished onto spoons we had stolen from the aforementioned cafeteria the year before.

I did, however, begin doing yoga with one of my roommates. We started out practicing in a church basement down the street from our house with a woman who was all long hair and soft voice. Most of the participants used straps and bolsters to get remotely close to the positions that me and my roommate – at least thirty years younger than most of them – readily twisted ourselves into. And then, in our second year practicing together, we switched to an intense Ashtanga class, and prided ourselves on being able to do poses that would impress our friends at house parties.

Between my second and third years of university, I decided to take time off to travel. I spent a month volunteering in an orphanage in Romania, and then in September, I jetted off to Australia for eight months.

Because reinvention had always been the name of the game for me, I had sincerely hoped that I would return from Australia tanned, *glowing* (always glowing), and, obviously, much, much thinner. Also, I decided I would be free of the face full of adult acne that I had begun to develop that year. Somehow. I had no *actual plan* as to how this would happen. My sense of that time in my life was that despite the fact that I had become more physically active, I *still* hadn't actually truly connected the notion of what it might take to lose weight with the outcome of having a thinner body: it's not as though I got on the airplane with an exercise plan or a diet strategy.

I realize now that this was something unique about my weight loss journey. I wonder, sometimes, if it has something to do with the fact that I was, growing up in a small town in the 80s and 90s, still blessedly unaware of the rampant exercise and diet culture that was raging around

me. Though the women that surrounded me "ate like birds," I never re-
member actually trying to restrict my own calorie intake. And exercise for
exercise's sake, at least until my later teenage years, was, in my perception,
judged by others as something I would only do if I hated my body. Which
I wanted to deny at all costs.

Although I can see it now, I didn't then: I held all this loathing for my physical appearance for so, so many years, and yet the extent of my efforts to *change anything* ended at the occasional new outfit or hairstyle during one of my many reinventions. Looking back, I think this is because I was in such deep denial of my self-hatred that it was impossible for me to diet or exercise, lest I have to admit to myself that I wanted to change myself.

I can't say whether this was a blessing or a curse. The result is that I spent many of my formative years loathing my weight but not actually doing anything to change those feelings. My denial spared me the potential harm of an eating disorder, or the toll that adolescent yo-yo dieting would have taken on my body. I feel as though I must have been intelligent and resourceful enough to discover any number of ways to shed weight, *and yet I didn't.*

As a result, I returned from Australia fairly *untransformed* and *unreinvented,* at least physically. I had, certainly, had some important experiences while there: I had a modicum of spending money from waitressing and teaching swimming lessons while I was there, and I found that there were more beautiful clothes for larger bodies available in Australia than there were in Canada. So I bought a few nice outfits. I bought my first bikini, a swimsuit so flattering that I actually *still* have the bottoms, almost twenty years later, somewhat see-through though they are now. I went topless for the first time (and sunburned my boobs). I had a couple of intimate experiences with men in a way I hadn't until that point in my life. The idea that I could be attractive to members of the opposite sex began to dawn on me, for the *very first* time in my life, at the ripe old age of 21. That is, until the first of many formative experiences happened at the hands of a man: someone I had picked up and "snogged" at a bar one night left me on the doorstep of my hostel saying, "if only you weren't a little bit fat and didn't have all that acne, you'd be perfect."

Scorched.

And *found out*. Someone *else* had noticed my fat body, and judged it as such.

Though I had battled with my weight my entire life, most of the negativity I had around my physical appearance had been, aside from the Meat Arms and Fat Witch Incidents, isolated to the space between my own two ears, and my *stories of people's perceptions of me,* but not, necessarily, their *actual perceptions.*

Perhaps it was this that allowed me to be in denial for so long. I never got a "talking to" from a doctor about losing weight. No one had ever really *told* me that I was less than or incapable or undeserving because I was fat, *except for me.*

But here it was. Someone noticed that which I had spent a vast majority of my time hoping they wouldn't.

Yeah, I was fat. And not only that, according to him: I would be *perfect,* if only I wasn't.

When I returned from Australia, something had happened among my university friends.

It had become cool to exercise.

Like, for exercise's sake. The stories and shame I had carried all my life about being caught exercising and judged for being fat, or for acknowledging I *was* fat and doing something to remedy that, evaporated. All of a sudden, my girlfriends were heading to the track to run laps in the mornings, or going to the university gym's yoga studio over lunch hours. It had become socially acceptable — even cool — to exercise. Now, it wasn't a sign that I was dissatisfied with my body and wanted to lose weight but rather just an overall indication of my desire to be healthy, just like my friends.

That summer, I began to run. Other than the triathlon I had done a couple years before, I had never really run. I started out running laps around the soft turf of the university soccer field late, late at night with a friend that I was working with at a residential summer school for teens. We would do a couple laps around the track and feel quite satisfied with ourselves. I do recall thinking, at the time: "This exercise thing is not too bad. It's kind of fun. I think I will continue to build this habit...and then I wonder if I might be able to shift my eating habits and....lose weight."

It was the first time this had really occurred to me, the first time that I had a bit of a *plan* to change my body. To, hopefully, ease my dissatisfaction with the way it looked.

When the Fall came, I began to run laps at the indoor track. I brought my portable CD player and listened to Bif Naked yell "I love myself today, not like yesterday!" I ran to the feminist moaning of my Hole album, and to the upbeat folk rock of Ani Difranco. I ran three days a week, flying around the track. By summer, running felt like freedom (*a feeling that I hadn't connected to before, or since*).

Then I managed to get a hold of the Points Guide for Weight Watchers. Both my mom and my sister were on the program, and so I thought I'd try my hand.

It worked.

The Big Loss

By the winter of that year, I had probably lost about 20 pounds. I say "probably" because, as a poor off-campus university student, I didn't have access to a scale during this time. I actually don't think I even knew what I weighed to begin with: in fact, interestingly, during *all* the years previous that I had wrestled with my weight, I can probably count the number of times I ever actually stepped on a scale.

My Weight Watchers experience is hallmarked by a few key memories. They all revolved around food — no surprise there. I remember feeling hungry after eating dinner. Often. I remember laying on my couch on my back after classes one day and feeling my hipbones rise up higher than my belly fat, for the first time in my life. I remember running, which always felt amazing. I felt strong. I walked everywhere. I also remember Cheat Nights. This was when myself and all of my friends would get together and eat EVERYTHING we wanted while watching Thursday night TV. I remember when Thursday Night Cheat Night began to extend to the rest of the day, too. I remember being really hungry and eating an entire sleeve of soda crackers carefully spread with peanut butter and honey with my roommate one night. I remember, one Cheat Night, having received a massive bar of chocolate for Valentine's Day from my mother, and wanting to eat more of it than I thought was socially acceptable in front of my peers. I remember sneaking into the kitchen during commercial breaks and eating square after square of it, being conscious that I finished chewing and sucking the chocolate from my teeth before I re-emerged into the room where my friends were, lest I be caught pigging out.

As I was digging into my History Experiment, I found some old journals from this time in my life, and, looking back at them with a different lens now, I see some deeply telltale signs of very disordered eating. I was probably at greater risk for developing an eating disorder than I could appreciate at the time. The risk factors certainly were there, not least of which were my Type A, controlling tendencies. Rather than journaling about what was happening in my life, my journal was more of a daily log of my intake and calories burned, along with the occasional diatribe about exams or boys. I ate shockingly little food: a small package of instant oatmeal with one tablespoon of raisins for breakfast, maybe a package of Mr. Noodles with steamed vegetables for lunch; I'd let myself have half a

frozen banana drizzled with melted peanut butter or two graham wafers
smeared with honey for dessert.

But oh, I remember the comments:

"Wow, you've really lost weight!"

"You look fabulous!"

"You seem to be someone who is really comfortable in your own skin" — this, from a new colleague at the time who hadn't witnessed my lifelong struggle with my weight. I won't forget her words: it was as if I had successfully donned the mask of self-acceptance by appearing more societally accept-able in my physical form.

"You lost all this weight in the healthy way, right?" — this, from my best guy friend. I won't forget his words, either. I scoffed at the time, and I now realize that he was expressing true concern for the rapidity with which I had transformed.

I bought new clothes.

Buying clothes was actually *fun*. I suddenly felt like I actually *belonged* among my peer group, who were, almost with-out exception, petite, fit women. I could *almost* fit into some of *their clothes*, thereby earning myself a place among that time-ho-noured university student tradition of sharing everything in each other's closets. The latter was a truly special occurrence for me: this was something that I had never been able to take part in in all my formative years, and I always felt deeply left out because of it. The experience of aloneness that I had always felt as a result of my weight began to dissipate.

That Spring Break, six of us took a trip to Cuba together, a vacation that would prove to be one of my favourite experiences of my university years.

I had lost enough weight that I was actually looking forward to spending a week in my bathing suit on the beach with my petite, fit friends.

I bought a bikini. It looked good. I regularly put it on and danced in front of the mirror.

I looked back at the pictures of myself from that holiday and yes, I did look great. At this point, after about a twenty pound weight loss, I was a fit but curvy woman, still with hips and thighs. I definitely still had the three characteristic (and, I thought, large) belly rolls that I had come to familiarize myself with over all my years of living in my body, but they were smaller. At the time, though, I couldn't see that. I lived with an experience of somehow both loving my body — probably fuelled by the positive feedback I was receiving from others — and still thinking it was too big.

The other thing that happened during this time in my life, shortly after we returned from Cuba, was that I started to attract men in a way that I hadn't before. This was a total first for me: I had, up until this point, hardly dated. My experience with members of the opposite sex was decidedly limited. I believe that there was some part of me that couldn't believe that I was truly "thin enough" or even attractive at all until I had earned the approval of a guy. I went on a few dates during this time, and I actually had the confidence to do a bit of online dating.

(For me, this took the motherlode of confidence: I didn't perceive online dating as being a safe place for me to hide my appearance, but rather a strangely commercialized experience whereby I had to describe the goods — me — in a way that would sell. After having the confidence to highlight my strengths, I then had to DELIVER. The "goods" had to be as good as they sounded in my online profile).

I had stopped actually actively *losing* weight by this time, and had settled out at around 145 pounds: I finally slinked into the campus doctor's office and weighed myself. I was both shocked I still weighed "so much" and in awe of all I had accomplished. Knowing my weight helped me to then formulate a "goal," which was to be 135 pounds. That's how much both my best friends weighed, and because of this, to me this seemed *normal.* Now, nothing would be quite perfect until I had lost that extra ten pounds. But, I returned to a state of not knowing exactly how to accomplish that: I was already doing everything I thought I could with diet and exercise, and I was at a loss as to what could be next. Thankfully, some intuition or inner wisdom or something couldn't allow me to truly starve myself, or to resort to more extreme methods. I had always been too much of a lover of food — too attached to my own sustenance — to be able to limit my eating in that way. I decided to stop counting Weight Watchers points: I knew inherently that that wasn't a long term game plan — at least not for me. My lifestyle was active and healthy.

That's when I met E. At this time, I was as fit as I had ever been. I was training for a triathlon again — this time the

Olympic distance event back in my hometown. As compared to my somewhat half-assed effort preparing for my first, sprint distance triathlon, this time I truly was training: I ran, swam and cycled almost every day of the week. I had gotten a job at a local scuba diving shop which was a ten kilometre bike ride away from my apartment. I did this commute every day and on my one "rest" day, I did a home yoga practice. I was scuba diving regularly, carrying hundreds of pounds worth of gear around like it was nothing.

E loved this. He loved my long, blonde ponytail. He moved in. He was my first "real" boyfriend.

And image mattered *a lot* to him. He was gorgeous, and a gym rat. He came from a ludicrously wealthy family who were also very caught up in appearances. We went to the gym together, and he taught me how to lift weights. He had a habit of rollerblading around our neighbourhood with his shirt off, leaving a trail of drooling women in his wake. He did not believe in bacon.

I found out later that literally not a *single* one of my friends or family liked him, but at the time I believed he was the ultimate affirmation of my own attractiveness and desirability. If I could snag him, I was *finally beautiful enough and thin enough to have been deemed worthy not just of a guy, but of a really gorgeous guy at that.*

But I see now that there were many ways in which I was not worthy, at least to him. E's mother took me shopping one fall day, and bought me thousands of dollars worth of clothes in an effort I now interpret as being about making me look so-

43

cially acceptable; allowed to cavort with her son. There was a time, shortly after that, at the family's cottage over Thanksgiving when he told me, as I stepped out of the shower, that I would be "perfect if it weren't for my belly fat."

That protrusion of my lower abdomen — a motherly shape I wore long before I became a mother — was under attack again. By another man.

I was deeply hurt.

But, as always, I felt so much shame at being ashamed of my body. I idealized body confidence and therefore *not* feeling confident about my body was deeply shameful. And so I couldn't really vocalize my hurt, for fear of stripping back a layer of shame to find yet more underneath.

And, technically, through all this time, I *was* still fat. I carried fat on my body, despite being incredibly fit and eating carefully. Not "fat on my body" as in a slight paunch or a love handle, no: I truly was curvy. There was a roundness to my belly that would not go away, a breadth to my swimmer's shoulders that came with extra weight around my chest. I have come to realize that I was probably always meant to be this shape, but at the time I could not understand *for the life of me* why I didn't look — *couldn't* seem to look — like my peers.

E left me. I thought we were going to get married and have babies, and he had other plans, it turns out. We had planned a trip around the world together, starting with several months in Australia, and he left without me. I, left to finish the final exams of my university degree, did so, drove thousands of

kilometres to my childhood home with all my worldly posses-
sions packed into my SUV, and made the decision to head out
on the trip anyway, without him. But not, in true twenty-some-
thing style, without first heading to the little town on the east
coast of Australia where he had since settled to see if we could
reconcile our differences.

We couldn't. He was seeing someone else, who he eventually married. He left the little town of Byron Bay that had
been his home and would become mine for a while. I stayed on,
finding work as a scuba guide in exchange for rent, and I griev-
ed.

Glowing

Despite the heartbreak that started it all, my time in Byron Bay was to become one of the most cherished times in my
life. I would wake at 4:30 every other morning, slip into my
running clothes, and run powerfully up to the lighthouse to
watch the early morning waves. I would fly down that hill, arms
outstretched, feeling as free as I ever have. I returned in time to
eat breakfast and have a cup of tea, and begin preparing the
6:30a.m. dive boat's departure. I hauled scuba tanks over my
head and oiled boat engines in my bikini top, with my wetsuit
arms wrapped around my waist. I spent my afternoons napping
in my hammock or occasionally swimming the length of the
local beach.

There's a photo of me from that time that I still look
back on fondly: my hair is waist-length and bleached from the

sun, my skin darkly tanned and *glowing*, I am healthy, and so, so utterly happy.

Glowing, at last.

These years, from the time I began losing weight with Weight Watchers to this time in Byron Bay, remained, in the more-than-a-decade that has passed since, the Time that I always wanted to somehow return to. Remember when I was that happy, with myself and my body? If only I could get back to that weight, I would be that happy again (right?). If only I still lived that lifestyle. If only, if only, if only…

Those feelings have caused me to return to Weight Watchers and various forms of calorie counting many times since, and I've never been able to reclaim that experience again.

I spent the remainder of that year travelling around New Zealand, Southeast Asia and India. In New Zealand, I got work slinging lattes and serving French pastries in a patisserie, and that ended the era of glow, for me. I ate and ate and ate. I snuck pieces of fudge from the glass pastry case when no one was looking, and I made sure to come home with ALL the day-old pastries to share with my roommates, and then I didn't. Share, that is. I licked fondant from spatulas and tasted my first Croquembouche. I walked everywhere and swam at the local pool but it didn't matter: I gained and gained and gained, and by the time I headed on the South Asian portion of my adventure, my preference was to wear Thai fisherman pants and scarves to hide my growing body. The cheap milkshakes and Pad Thai on this leg of the journey didn't help, nor did the more sedentary nature of my lifestyle. I walked everywhere, but gyms and swimming pools were few and far between. When I ran, I attracted a lot of unwanted attention for being a white chick in Spandex, so I stopped doing that, too. I rented bicycles often and pedalled around, but it wasn't enough to counteract the effects of long days of travel and a plethora of new, novel and incredibly cheap restaurant foods to try.

When a friend suggested I try eating regular tofu instead of deep fried tofu with my daily Pad Thai, I felt like maybe I had overdone it. It was as though I, and my body, had responded to the years of Weight Watchers-induced deprivation with a six month-long binge. When I returned home from the trip and unpacked all the clothes I'd left behind, it was confirmed. Nothing fit. I had gotten fat again.

And so I decided to start training for a marathon.

Striving, Football and Pain

I'm not sure why training for a marathon became the Next Most Obvious Choice, but that's what I did. I spent a couple of months after my travels living with my parents, and worked my way up to twelve kilometre-long runs. It was painful. Literally. Running hurt in a way that it hadn't before: I had hip pain and shin splints. *I pushed through it.* When I returned to live in the city where I'd gone to university, I resumed my old scuba diving job, biking sometimes hundreds of kilometres a week to and from work. My relationship with exercise was reignited, once more.

Training for a marathon invited me into an entirely new relationship with food, though: one of food as fuel. I remember my first real experience of this quite clearly. I had just come home from a twenty-five kilometre run, and I was on my period. I felt a bone-deep exhaustion that was almost indescribable, and I knew, intuitively, that I needed meat. Iron. Protein. I went to the grocery store and filled my cart: ham, fish, steak, ground beef — everything you could possibly imagine. My diet up until that point had been largely vegetarian, mostly out of financial necessity and a general feeling of ambivalence about meat.

When I was training, I was able to eat anything I wanted. I was connected to a physical sensation of hunger a great portion of the time, as one can imagine would happen after doing vast amounts of physical activity every day.

I noticed it.

I freakin' THRIVED in it.

I had a TOTAL JOY about eating that stemmed primarily from a loss of the shame that came with it for me.

In fact, the presence of that shame was never so obvious as when it had suddenly disappeared.

I ate what I wanted and when I wanted. My extreme levels of physical activity allowed me to give myself *true* permission — not the overindulgent permissiveness accompanied by debilitating guilt and self-hatred — but a *true and total permission* to eat whatever the hell I wanted.

What I ate was never "all bad" — whatever that means. I still cooked myself healthy meals, ate out only occasionally, and rarely ever had fast food. But if I wanted cookies, I ate cookies. I never told myself to wait until the next meal, or until morning, or until next week, or *until I deserved it.*

I lost a bit of the weight while training for the marathon that I had put on during my travels, but my body certainly still clung to quite a bit of it, as well. But my perspective had changed: I had tapped into that sense of my own *ability* again, that same feeling that got me interested in moving my body more in the first place. I loved the feeling of being able to eat to fuel my body and to have that food be just about anything I wanted because my body was working so hard all the time. I wanted more.

Shortly after finishing the race, I was thrust into yet another period of what I now recognize as overexercising. I had the predictable slump post-race, not sure what to do with myself when I didn't have to train for hours on end, and craving that near-daily feeling of accomplishment and pride in myself. So, I joined a women's tackle football team for their inaugural season in my city.

Deciding to play on a team brought along with it all kinds of interesting feelings that I could connect back to my days of sitting on the dodgeball court in elementary school, being afraid of being hit by a ball. It was one thing to do the solo activities that I had become accustomed to — running, swimming, cycling — but another thing entirely to play on a team.

It turns out, though, I loved it. I loved training hard with other women who were just as dedicated to conditioning their bodies for the game as I was. I loved the badass factor of it all, and I felt surprisingly thrilled about smashing into people and connecting with an aggression that I rarely had an outlet for in my day-to-day life. As much as playing, I loved the *idea* of playing, and I loved what I thought others must think of me now that I was a *football player*.

The thing I loved best about football, I think, was that there was a special place for every *body* on the team. Unlike just about any other sport I know, a football team is one of the most physically diverse sports teams out there. It's not just about being able to *accommodate* people of different sizes — in football, certain body types are *specialized* for certain roles. They're *desired*. The tiny, fast women were free safeties and quarterbacks; the solidly built, fit, thick-thighed former rugby players belonged as running backs; the tall, larger women made a perfect offensive line, and I belonged as a medium-built, moderately fast, tough-as-nails linebacker. I *belonged*. And so did everyone else on the team, not regardless of their size, but *because* of their size. To me, this was revelatory.

That summer, I also trained for a half-marathon, running a personal best time — hitting my goal of an under-2 hour race — before heading straight to a two hour football practice. While hitting a quarterback particularly hard, I sprained the ligaments in my ankle.

This was the first of many injuries to come. The lexicon of pain was starting to become familiar to me, as was a routine of regularly visiting physiotherapists, massage therapists and chiropractors.

In addition to finding football that summer, I found the man who would become my husband. We met while I was working at the scuba shop: I taught him how to dive, and fell in love with his beautiful blue eyes and his gentle nature. And he *loved* that I played football, too. As with any courtship, my regular workout routine went a little pear-shaped, and I spent lots of time snuggling and driving back and forth to his house so that I could be snuggled. And, as with many courtships, I began eating like a man. He didn't ascribe to my almost-vegetarian, tofu-loving ways, and I began to *allow myself* things — takeout Chinese food was a particular favourite — that were so far out of my schema of *Things I Would Eat* that I wouldn't have even considered them *on a binge.*

By the following summer we had bought a house together and adopted a dog, and I had gained what I felt was an uncomfortable amount of weight. When I returned to football that season, I found myself playing on the offensive line more often than as a linebacker (read: I was bigger and slower than the year before), and early in the season in a gory debacle on the field, I dislocated my left knee. I spent the remainder of the summer almost entirely immobile, and the weight continued to pile on.

This injury solidified my place among the *injured athletes of the world*, and along with it I carried a story of nearly constant pain and discomfort. An exercise therapist later theorized that I had "shocked" my body, after spending the large majority of my childhood fairly sedentary, my body had grown up the body of a sedentary person. When I began working it as hard as I did in the tiny span of time that I did, my body simply couldn't handle the strain.

My story of overexercising doesn't end there, though. Always craving another feather for my cap, the following winter I began to train to do a long distance swim from the province of New Brunswick to the province of Prince Edward Island. While I was at it, I also made the decision to climb Mount Kilimanjaro, three weeks after completing the swim. I spent hours and hours and hours swimming laps in the pool that winter, this time no stranger to the way that I had to shape my life around my training schedule, allowing long hours for post-training naps, and an enthusiastically-welcomed increase to my caloric intake. Just a few short months before I was to complete the swim, I threw my back out in the first episode of what would later be diagnosed as degenerative disc syndrome. I continued my training regimen, hobbling to the lake, bent at the waist at a nearly forty-five degree angle, my only relief from my constant pain being the moment gravity subsided when I stepped into the water.

And so, that summer, I certainly did achieve the feats of breaking a world record for the fastest swim across the Northumberland Strait, and I was lucky enough to fight through altitude sickness and summit Mount Kilimanjaro, but I tucked these feathers in my cap along with a great deal of pain, which I have continued to live with ever since.

This time in my life was also a time, I believe, of great exploration and some healing — but also the addition of some complexity — around food. Owning a home and being married somehow brought out the domestic goddess in me, and I became quite enamoured with cooking, and began to identify as a pretty serious foodie. It was at this time that I most deeply began to relate to food as a way to nurture and connect with others. I cooked multi-course Indian meals, perfected Italian risotto, and couldn't attend an occasion or hang out with friends without bringing some goodie or another. There were dinner parties and recipe exchanges and I loved every minute of it. There was healing in this as I started to see food as more than just calories that needed to be burned, as I had done in the years previous. But there was complexity to it too: it felt difficult to *stop* cooking and eating elaborate meals. I began to use food as my *primary* method of connecting and nurturing others — and myself — and then felt badly about indulging. My complex relationship with food continued to deepen.

Having Babies

They say

they're tiger stripes

or battle scars

I don't buy it.

They are rifts in my skin, wide canyons carved into my flesh

because I had to expand for you.

because I got to expand for you.

because I allowed myself to expand for you.

Though the skin of my thighs and breasts had been riven with stretch marks since puberty, those markings felt "normal" to me. All of my friends had them; they were a sign we were growing up, getting older, going through a rite of passage.

When I got my first stretch mark on my belly, it was a shock that would have me reaching down, lifting my shirt, and running my fingers over its silky presence absentmindedly through the day. At the time, I remember being surprised because though I had, perhaps, added some weight to my frame over the previous months, this red rivulet was proof that my expansion hadn't gone unnoticed. It couldn't be swept under the rug. There it was, objective proof that I

had let myself go

had porked up

needed to lose weight.

Naturally, right?

I kept a very close eye on that stretch mark as my pregnancy with my daughter progressed, several years later. It shifted position but, to my surprise and delight, I didn't grow any more of the telltale marks of motherhood.

If you'd asked me at the time, I would have sounded very *neutral* about the whole thing.

"Nope, didn't happen to me. I guess not everyone gets stretch marks."

"Yeah, I'm lucky."

"It must be my genes."

But I would later find out that I was more attached to my almost-smooth lower belly than I had originally realized.

After all, it was a part of my body that had been under scrutiny all too many times before.

After I had my daughter, breastfeeding and calorie counting and baby-wearing and a great many hikes in the woods brought me down to a size I hadn't seen since long before my pregnancy. When I returned to work, I bought an entirely new wardrobe.

I felt great.

One of my colleagues said, "Jessie, you're shrinking away!"

I took this as a compliment, and I basked in it.

Though my waistline had thickened slightly after pregnancy and changed the way my pants fit and how I felt wearing tight t-shirts, I felt fantastic about how I looked.

And I just had a baby.

I took more pride in that than I realized.

After I returned to work from my year of maternity leave, my daughter had a string of daycare-wrought illnesses that had at least one of our family down for the count at any given time for the next six months. It started with a stomach flu; what followed were innumerable cases of pinkeye, ear infections, and fever upon fever upon fever.

And so for six months, I rarely felt well. I went over three months without moving my body more than to simply go up and down the stairs of our house or to walk through the parking garage to my cubicle at work. I had no energy left at the end of a long day to cook a healthy meal. These months were, in essence, worse than those very early newborn months that I thought I had escaped from.

At the same time as all this was happening, I had started to deeply question my career choices. With a baby at home, I simply didn't have time for being unhappy in my career. I couldn't justify being away from her all day just to sit on in a cubicle feeling miserable. So I started some tiny experiments that allowed me to pursue some of the things I enjoyed the most, and one of these tiny experiments was a food blog. Like everything else in my life, I dove into that blogging experience with BOTH FEET. I was convinced that perhaps someone would "discover me" and my site would attract hundreds of thousands of visitors and I would be offered a cookbook deal and *that would be it*: I would be able to quit my job to become a full time food blogger. I DID do very well for myself with my food blog, scoring some really fun freelance food writing gigs and getting some attention for my writing, but mostly, I was writing three (THREE!) blog posts a week (this is literally un-heard of in the food blogging realm: each blog post takes hours and hours to develop, recipe test, write, and photograph) and I was getting really fat eating the food I had created.

I gained weight. More and more weight. I was amazed to feel parts of my body that just simply didn't exist before. I would continuously run my hands over my fleshed out hips that now created a cushion for me when I sat down, wide wide wide at the base. My arms had more flesh under the armpits and my chest more width around the ribcage, such that it felt strangely constricting around my heart sometimes. My stomach no longer had the three rolls that I had come to familiarize myself with over their longstanding presence in my life. In fact, I real-ized, after all those years of loathing those rolls, that three rolls is *better* than one, because one roll meant that the three I used to have had *filled in*.

As I would run my hands over these strange new parts of me, I felt like I was living in someone else's body.

I went to a naturopath, thinking that maybe my thyroid had become completely dysfunctional during my postpartum period, as happens to many new mothers. Sadly, tests revealed that no, I had just put on weight and, apparently, the only thing to be done was to get serious about vegetables.

There were salads for lunch that became famously enormous among my colleagues — piles upon piles of spinach and arugula and lettuce. There was a juice cleanse, at one point. I attempted to resume my old levels of physical activity. Unlike during my pre-kid life, this became the most challenging thing of all, and not due to my lack of motivation but rather the simple inability to find a time that I could get out the door without a tiny little accomplice.

Slowly, as my weight increased despite my efforts, I also became concerned about my ability to "keep up" in the physical endeavours I engaged in before. I found myself a little nervous to go for a run for fear my knees would hurt too much with my added heft. I feared that I would have become a slow swimmer or biker in the time since I had last enjoyed those sports. I worried that my larger stomach would get in the way of my favourite yoga poses. This was a new realization for me; a doubt in my own ability that I had never experienced before. Because exercise provided me not only with what I believed to be a more acceptable body but also a great portion of my self-esteem, this doubt plagued me.

I started to feel like *one of those people* that I had always been thankful I *hadn't been*: one of those women who was afraid to go on a hike for fear it would be too challenging.

This, like the wideness in my butt that I couldn't stop marvelling at (in the way of a bystander to a train wreck), felt like the experience of another person to me. Not me.

When my daughter was two and a half, my husband left on a six month deployment overseas.

No sooner had his ship left the harbour, my age-old fantasies of personal transformation came thundering back. I was awash in a dreamy image of me looking like a completely new (aka twenty pounds lighter) woman when he returned.

Having always somewhat blamed my poor husband for the weight gain that really began to skyrocket after I met him, I assumed this would be the perfect chance to get back to the tofu-scarfing, extremely active woman I was when we first started dating. Nevermind that I would be single parenting; in a way, I figured, not having to cook for an entire family and being able to make whatever foods I felt like was going to be the key to my successful weight loss this time around.

I had it all planned out, and then, after feeling particularly lightheaded and nauseous during the juice cleanse that was meant to kick the whole process off, I found out that I was pregnant again.

What ensued were many months of indomitable exhaustion and fierce hormone surges that had me unable to muster the energy or "give-a-shit factor" to eat anything other than takeout Lebanese. The time of my pregnancy that my husband was deployed was one of the darkest times of my life. I was deeply ashamed of my frustrated parenting of my daughter; I spent most evenings after she had gone to bed in a near-catatonic state in front of the television. This state of being couldn't have been farther from who I wanted and knew myself to be; like my widened hips and my physical inability, it felt like another person had taken over my existence.

Interestingly, and simultaneously, I felt fantastic about my body.

(None of this would be very interesting without a truly confusing juxtaposition, right?)

During both my pregnancies with each of my children, I felt like a damn goddess. I remember writing a poem in my journal while I was pregnant with my daughter about how amazing my incredibly pregnant body looked: belly round and taut, hips wide, breasts resting gloriously on the mound of my growing baby. I loved how I looked in my maternity clothes, and rocked fashions that felt truly "me." Lots of beautiful fabrics, layers, scarves, jewellery. I even found the audacity to wear some truly eclectic outfits amongst my austere-looking colleagues; I felt so amazing.

I don't think I felt this way because, as a doula, I have been socialized to see pregnant women's bodies as incredible works of art; I believe I felt this way about myself simply because of what I woke up and saw in the mirror every day. I loved the way I looked while I was pregnant.

My pregnancies were, as when I had trained for the marathon, a time in my life when I truly lost all judgment of the food I ate. I associated almost no guilt or misgivings or "shoulds" with my intake of nourishment. I was making a human, after all, and so I just didn't think about food that much, and I felt so much freer as a result. I noticed that I didn't notice. It was more than not *caring*; no, I just ate whatever I felt like and didn't feel badly about it. I gained the "appropriate" amount of weight for pregnancy and didn't think twice. It was one of the few times in my life when I wasn't completely wrapped up in management, control, and ultimate dissatisfaction with my body.

The freedom of this was tangible.

But the second time around, I got stretch marks. I suppose I wasn't miraculously genetically indisposed of them after all. My lower belly, that contested ground I had warred with my whole life, became full of stretch marks. They were thick and deep and they riveted and snaked their way across my most loathed physical feature.

I again ran my fingers over them like they belonged to somebody else.

But perhaps what's more important is that what happened during my pregnancies and births was something so much more than unlimited shawarmas without guilt. Even more than stretch marks, in fact.

What I witnessed in my body was the ability to be perfect and to *create* perfection in a vessel that I had spent the last thirty years quietly and daily scolding for *not* being perfect. Not in that *oh well nobody's perfect* kind of way; no — somewhere in me was a deeply held expectation that I should not look the way I looked, that I did not belong in the skin I was born in. That I was a thin person waiting to happen. This was a deeply, deeply held conviction that had almost never surfaced into words, but merely in my silent loathing and subsequent attempts to become acceptable to myself.

But here I was, a woman lucky enough to have gotten pregnant without difficulty, who carried two babies and *felt good doing it.* I created two perfect human beings with my body.

And then, somehow — and I still marvel at this — despite the systemic hatefulness I've geared toward my body my entire life, I was able to trust my body enough to birth. My work in the birth community has magnified just how incredible this is, because I see the myriad ways in which women, our culture and the institutions and systems of birth *distrust* women's bodies' innate ability to conceive, carry, birth and nurture babies. I have seen how deeply women embody that distrust, so much so that they don't believe they can birth without the assistance of the very institutions and systems of birth that have created the distrust they feel. Most women carry a deeply-held fear that their bodies will somehow do them wrong in the birth process: that they won't be able to handle the pain, that their baby will be too big or their hips too small, that they won't make enough milk to feed their babies. The systems within which they birth perpetuate and support those beliefs. And so we have created technology in the form of epidurals and operations and pretend breastmilk. So that *when* — and we assume it's a *when* and not an *if* — women's bodies fail them, we will have the technology to counteract that failure.

Though we trust Mother Nature's wise design in other ways — we do not try to prevent the tides or change the seasons or wish the blue of the sky away — we do not trust that women's bodies are meant to perform the very function that ensures the survival of our species. The very function that is required to uphold our knowledge of evolution and our understanding of why we're here and why we are the way we are.

Somehow, I didn't have doubts about my body's ability to birth. I consider this nothing short of miracle, really, and I am in awe and deep respect of other women who have come to know the same. We are a small but growing subculture. And so I birthed my babies without complication, births that were so powerful that they will forever impact my perceptions of what I am capable of. Which is to say….*anything*. And then I nursed both my babies for extended periods of time, and watched how my body created the very thing — the everything — they needed to survive in the world.

And yet, when the glow of pregnancy was over, I still could not truly *see*, in the rounds of my twice-expanded flesh, the ability to create and house life. I still could not *see* my physical self as a miracle, a miracle-maker. I could only see how my shape had become distorted by the perfect act of childbearing. How my breasts hung flatter and lower, how my abdomen, streaked with those stretch marks, protruded, how my arms and legs had thickened. I blamed the lack of time, the always-running-after-the-kids, no-time-to-work out. I blamed myself. I was filled with not-enoughness. Though I saw the effects of our cultural beliefs on women's experience of body-trust during birth, I was blind to the effects of that culture on my perceptions of my own physical worth in the world, despite or because of my motherhood.

During this phase of my life, a journal entry I wrote reads: *"This is unacceptable. I have a problem. I have a problem. I have a problem. This is not something that might be okay. This is not about my thyroid, not about getting older or being a mother. This is ON ME — and it's happened because I have ABNORMAL and DESTRUCTIVE eating habits that are hurting my body and my spirit. It's not okay, and I need to take responsibility for it, EVERY SINGLE MINUTE OF EVERY SINGLE DAY."*

When I look back on those words, scribbled so fiercely they left indentations on the following pages of my notebook, tears well in my eyes. They were words of disgust, shame and punishment, but also words of helplessness. How could I be such an intelligent, accomplished woman and yet *fail in the simple act of feeding myself, of keeping myself "healthy"?*

This experience of myself in my postpartum body was cemented with an ironic experience I had shortly after the birth of my son. At the time, there was a photo of a group of women breastfeeding that was going viral on the internet. It was being met with a healthy dose of controversy about women baring their bodies, about breastfeeding in general and specifically the sexualization of women's breasts and the appropriateness of extended breastfeeding. I decided to get a group of my mama friends together to take a similar photo. My intention was one of helping myself and others to find beauty in their postpartum shapes, to see themselves as beautiful in a photograph that was indeed beautiful, and to perhaps come to some level of acceptance. The photo turned out wonderfully, and I decided to write an article about the experience and submit it for publication on a wellness blog with several million readers. The article was accepted and went a little bit viral on that blog. What I wasn't prepared for, though, was the onslaught of other people's opinions about my body and those of the women I stood in the photo with. I thought that the article was irrefutably "feel-good" in nature, and would elicit all kinds of warm and fuzzy feelings. I was not expecting to have my every curve analyzed by a scrutinizing public, my choice of underwear berated, and to be told that if I would only *dedicate myself* to healthy living, I wouldn't be *so fat.*

Of the thousands of comments that poured in, I could only see the negative ones. To say I was shocked would have been the understatement of the year. To say that I was ashamed for having exposed my beautiful mama friends to this same kind of scrutiny couldn't even begin to describe my emotions. Like the proverbial train wreck I couldn't turn my attention away from, the comments kept pouring in, and I couldn't seem to rationalize that they were being made by horrible, evil, troll-like people with big problems of their own who couldn't help but put other people down from the safety of the uncensored internet. Intellectually, this is how I *wanted* to react to this response, and this is how others told me I *should* react, but I can say with certainty that those comments affected me profoundly, and for a long time. They set in motion this deep sense of discomfort with my postpartum body, whereas before the photo, I had somewhat succeeded in being gentler on myself for having just recently given birth and for living in a body that looked like it.

Something happened after that photo, and I can't help but think that some universal wisdom was at work, propelling me toward a deeper inquiry in my relationship with my physical self.

Denial

When I began writing this book, two years postpartum and thirty-five years into my life, I felt as though I was still in deep denial of my body, and began to realize that perhaps I always had been. I would run my hands over my hips when I sat in a hard chair, and noticed how they expanded outward to form a cushion for the rest of me in a way they didn't before. The extra pounds I had always carried had never quite spilled out beside me like they did now. When I crossed my legs, one over the other, I would run my fingers along the dimpling I now have in my thighs. That was new to me, too. Though I had always had stretch marks, they had never created a cratered landscape like my thighs have now. I grew skin tags between my breasts during my pregnancies that have never fallen off but that aren't large enough to be removed. I ran my fingers over them regularly, too, feeling as though I had a different landscape than I used to.

I have become new terrain.

Every day in those early postpartum months, I had an intense experience of not recognizing the body I lived in anymore. It didn't feel like it used to or look like it used to, and my hands and fingers were compulsively drawn to try to make sense of this new physicality. While many women have a hateful dialogue with themselves when they look in the mirror, mine was neutral, as though I could not direct sharp words at myself and the way I looked because this *could not possibly be me.* My lack of acceptance ran so deep that I could not even fathom that what I saw in the mirror was actually *me.*

I came to realize, as my history experiment wound to a close, that though this journey was intended to be about self-acceptance, body respect, and maybe even body love, perhaps what I wanted the most was just to feel like myself again. To feel like I belonged in my body, and that *my body belonged in the world.*

***

With the nuggets of revelation about my history of relating to and living in my body uncovered, I began to feel drawn to explore some more small and do-able actions — more tiny experiments — that I believed would help me to feel like myself again, help me to feel more at home in my own skin, more accepting of my body.

The first of these experiments were deeply pragmatic, and very small. When I began them, what I realized I needed most was to simply care for myself. To identify the very basic needs that I had, and meet them. Because I started these experiments at my lowest low point, they focused less on coming to terms with the fatness of my body, and more on simply tending to my body with the things it required. Perhaps it was like the Maslow's Hierarchy of Body Love: start with the basics — brush your teeth and drink some water — and then think about the bigger stuff. Also, starting with these things felt safe, to me, and very doable in the face of one of the gnarliest "problems" — my unacceptance of my body — I've ever battled.

The Basic Hygiene Experiment

As a mom of two kids, my journey toward self-acceptance needed to start *before* square one. At eighteen months postpartum with my second child I had started feeling like I was ready to turn some attention toward myself again, but I wasn't even ready to start with physical activity and healthy eating, which is how I *thought* I might begin this journey.

No.

Because my pits stunk.

My teeth were furry.

My hair was a stringy mass of wayward cowlicks on my head.

Somehow, the things that were, at one point, automatic elements of my personal maintenance — we're not even talking "self care" here, people, just basic hygiene — had fallen by the wayside. I often would fall asleep while putting my young son to bed, or would put him to sleep in the baby carrier, rendering it impossible for me to lean over his sleeping body to spit toothpaste into the sink. And so my toothbrushing routine became relegated to the mornings.

Only.

My husband would leave for work before the kids and I were awake, and so for a long time I rarely had a chance to shower before leaving the house in the morning. Not without risking having both kids electrocute themselves / drown / fall down the stairs. For a while I rocked the kind of haircut that looked pretty good when I rolled out of bed in the morning, and I washed my hair infrequently enough that in fact it was less oily and needed to be washed less often. But I grew my locks out a bit, and dyed them a shade of blonde that made my naturally oily hair look even gnarlier at the end of the day, let alone after a night of tossing and turning beside a nursing toddler.

And also, something about my pregnancy with my son changed something about my physiology. I have no actual scientific evidence to back up this phenomenon, but I do know that, among other changes, I became a stinky person. No amount of deodorant — lady-style, men's, homemade or all-natural — could conquer the smell of my armpits.

Too much information, perhaps; but I'm endeavouring for full disclosure here.

It became clear to me that there was no way I could even dream of self-acceptance and self-love when I was finding it hard to prioritize myself enough to just *stay clean.*

So, for the first couple of months — *yes, couple of months* — of my tiny experiments, I just tried to get regular showers and not have furry teeth.

Ambitious, indeed.

But my intentions did require a bit of planning. I had to make sure I was awake early enough in the mornings to have a shower while my husband watched the kids. Our bedtime routines changed, gradually over time, so that I was unencumbered and unattached to a baby when it came time for me to turn in for the night, and so I could take the couple of minutes that I needed to brush my teeth.

I even started dry-brushing my skin in the mornings before my shower. This practice is supposed to be detoxifying, and I have no idea if it really is, but just the act of spending a few moments doing something that *might be* detoxifying felt like a move in the right direction for me.

I sought out some professional advice when it came to my armpits. I had long since tried *everything,* and decided that there was a distinct possibility that the root of the problem had something to do with what was *inside* my body, trying to get out.

Via my super-stinky pits.

I used a few naturopathic remedies, increased my probiotic and water intake, and went to get a lymph-draining massage. I changed deodorants One Last Time.

And strangely, the smell went away. I was expecting a fight, but alas. Along with it, and with the addition of a stronger personal hygiene game that was not so easily high-jacked by the demands of my two kids, I began to feel...human again. Like I was on a level playing field with all the other people who managed to have showers in the morning. Like I could look those people, and everyone else for that matter, in the eye, knowing my hair wasn't a wonky, greasy mess, and that I could hug them, if I wanted, without overwhelming them with the smell of my pits.

The Hydration Experiment

The other painfully basic task ahead of me when it came to nourishing my body was simply getting more hydration. I used to be one of those people who was attached at the hip (literally, with a carabiner) to her Nalgene bottle, faithfully sipping back at least two litres of water a day. Somewhere, among the losses of other great habits and gains of several unhelpful ones, I stopped drinking very much water at all. I found myself getting so thirsty that I would crave something different than water — most usually juice or something fizzy. I was also generally so tired that I would consume a great number of cups of tea and coffee in a day — to wake myself up, to ritualize and find comfort in tasks I found mundane or undesirable, to connect with friends, or just to pass the time.

So I decided to simply add back in the habits of hydration that had kept me well-watered in the past. I started drinking hot lemon water and honey in the morning alongside my cup of tea, which I tried to keep to one large but single mug over the course of the day. I also started simply filling up the water bottle that I had always had sitting on my desk when I was working, and taking the time to actually leave my office and refill it when it was empty. I started drinking tap water at a medium temperature so that I could drink more at one sitting.

Though these seemed like small steps, everything I read about getting more water into my body showed that it would be beneficial. I liked to think about how my plants respond to being watered once a week — they plump up (like, in the good, adorable way), and truly come back to life. They are more vibrant and often will start or continue to flower as a result. I felt like hydrating more would bring a bit more vibrancy into my body, too, and that maybe I could begin to turn to hydration as a way to stay awake and find energy through the day, or to get curious about whether my hunger was true hunger or actually something else. I'm proud to report that on a particularly exhausting day a short while ago, I thought first of water as a way to wake up and keep going, rather than brewing another cup of coffee.

I don't have anything to prove this, but I'd also like to think all this water is flushing crap out of my system — both literally, physically, and potentially metaphorically.

I noticed, as I contemplated my hydration experiment, that choosing to drink more water was, for me, a much less value-laden decision than choosing to restrict my eating, as I had done in the past. I have no complex stories about water. *"It's good for me so I'll drink more of it."* No problem, end of story. It was a "simple" problem with what turned out to be some very simple solutions that came in the form of creating a few new habits and remembering a few old ones.

Interestingly, though, with every sip of cool liquid from every receptacle I filled, I actually found myself creating a new story about water. It was a positive story, a story of self-care. Instead of thoughtlessly chugging back my daily hydration, I would simply notice that I was hydrating myself, and I would equate the act of sipping water as being in service to myself. I found myself reaching for water when I was a little frustrated or needed a moment to think, or was feeling tired or anxious.

Water was an easy place to start — the act of drinking it had only positive connotations for me, linked directly to my well-being. I could truly nourish myself with water, and so I started being mindful of times when I needed that kind of nourishing, and meeting those needs with water.

The Sleep Experiment

In the past few years, I've been burning the midnight oil building my business while working full time and mothering (as well as, you know, trying to remain a not only functioning but somewhat joyful human). I am a morning person, and as I contemplated how I might find time for myself and my writing while keeping up with everything else, I decided to start waking up at 4a.m. to write. At the same time, though, I was finding it difficult to make a choice between the early mornings that quickly became a sacred and nourishing time for me, and spending my evenings attempting to have quality time with my husband, zoning out in front of the TV, or doing other things for the sheer pleasure of them. And so, for about two years, I simply didn't make the choice.

It meant that I was getting, on average, about four hours of sleep per night.

The crazy thing was: I was convinced that it wasn't affecting me. I started wondering if maybe there was a broader spectrum of normal to the eight hours nightly that "normal" people supposedly need. My energy was great, I only ever drank one caffeinated beverage per day, and I never felt tired.

When I started to see a naturopath about my stinky pits, though, I couldn't convince her that this sleepless lifestyle was actually healthy for me; that there was nothing "wrong" with me. I could have been miffed by her distrust in my intuition about what felt good for me, but because she was a friend and because I like experiments, I decided I would try sleeping seven hours a night for a week. Just to see what happened.

I felt better.

I thought I felt great with four hours of sleep, but with seven, I felt better.

I won't call it a total *win,* on my naturopath's part, but as a result of this experiment, I did decide to change the shape of my life and my priorities to make sure I always got at least seven hours of sleep per night.

Now, even when life feels tremendously chaotic, not unlike my water guzzling, I can rely on my ability to get a nourishing night's sleep as the tiniest — albeit quite impactful — form of self-care.

The Adornment Experiment

"I want to live the most vividly decorated temporary life that I can. I don't just mean physically; I mean emotionally, spiritually, intellectually. I don't want to be afraid of bright colours, or new sounds, or big love, or risky decisions, or strange experiences, or weird endeavours, or sudden changes, or even failure." — *Elizabeth Gilbert*

As I began, through my tiny experiments, to meet some of my body's most basic human needs in a better way, I started to think about how I might continue to find more of the fledgling nourishment of self-care and self-acceptance I had started to feel.

The Adornment Experiment actually started, inadvertently, months before I ever conceived of embarking on this journey or writing this book, with the purging of my maternity clothes. I hadn't been wearing them *that* often since having my son two years ago: no, what I *had* been wearing, though, was a lot of elastic waist-banded pants. But if I did have to don a pair of jeans or dress pants to jazz up my appearance a little bit, on came the maternity clothes. They fit me beautifully and were wonderfully forgiving, and allowed me to "dress up" in a pinch, but the truth is that they were making me actually *look* pregnant.

Also, a note: as I wrote this, I noticed some self-shaming around the idea of STILL wearing maternity clothes, and also about wearing elastic waistbanded pants. As I noticed myself thinking this, I thought:

now what in sweet hell is wrong with wearing clothes that are COM-FORTABLE?

I also went about almost entirely ridding myself of the clothes I had been harbouring from years — and sizes — past in the hopes that I would one day fit them again. I had drawers and drawers of these clothes. There were a beautiful series of dress pants I bought at the Gap when I got my first Real Job out of my graduate degree. There were *a lot* of things that I wore when I went through my Weight Watchers years. And there were a good few articles of clothing that held great nostalgia for me: a pair of board shorts that I had owned since my first trip to Australia in 2001, which had somehow fit me through many of my weight fluctuations and had always looked good (but finally, I had to admit, no longer afforded me that pleasure). This was a pretty sentimental process: I had kept those clothes in a somewhat sick combination of motivation and punishment. I would try them on, periodically, and feel completely awful about the fact that I had "allowed myself" to *get so big,* so big that I couldn't fit into these beautiful, favourite clothes. But when I tried them on I would immediately also become motivated to fit into them again. So back in the chest of drawers they would go, and I would make promises and set goals and intentions for what I would do *this time* to finally Lose The Weight, to finally be able to fit back into my treasured clothes.

Getting rid of all of these clothes felt cathartic, and it felt accepting. It felt a *little bit* like acknowledging that I had a *new body.* That new body, even if could miraculously return to the same weight as I was before having children, was shaped differently now, and might never quite *look* the same in the clothes I so cherished. And the part of me that *still* harboured the desire to lose weight said "It's okay to get rid of these…you can always buy new clothes." But losing the ability to bench-mark *where I had been*, size-wise, felt a little risky to me. It felt like I might be giving myself *permission* to just *let myself go*, now that I had no way of knowing *how far gone I truly was.* I had lost the ability to punish myself for the amount of weight I had gained, to feel sad for the body I used to have (which still, I *always must remember,* was dissatisfying to me at the time).

This showed me that the underlying feelings I had about my body were still there: they weren't about to be solved with some new outfits.

Regardless, I went about purchasing a new, small, and very versatile wardrobe of clothing that looked and felt good on me. I developed for myself a sort of uniform that always looked good, no matter how I was feeling that day. I purchased:

Plain black leggings, a pair of comfortable Lululemon pants, a pair of black skinny jeans, and a pair of grey linen dress pants to be worn with

A few drapey, colourful, patterned tank tops that could be paired with

Either my go-to favourite IceBreaker wrap, a denim overshirt or an unbuttoned black and white plaid shirt

Always a scarf

For the summer, I paired my tanks with a solid few pairs of comfortable shorts, both dressy and casual, and a handful of long flowing dresses and skirts.

I also tried to make a point of adorning myself in other ways, too. I have a massive collection of jewellery that I adore wearing. I always like to have a watch and a few bracelets on, I rotate out some simple earrings on a regular basis, and the occasional necklace. I very often dab some essential oils between my breasts and behind my ears: my favourite is a rose and geranium oil mixture that was gifted to me by a Reiki Master, but sometimes I go with something a little heavier and more grounding, like Black Spruce or Patchouli, or feminine, spicy or energizing, like jasmine, cassia or bergamot. Lavender and spearmint are for days when I need a bit of a pick- me-up.

On a day-to-day basis, once I had mastered showering, hydrating and keeping my stinky pits at bay, I started to feel fairly "put together," or at least like I could achieve that state of being fairly efficiently if I wanted to: no fretting in front of the mirror, trying on one thing after the next, grabbing at my fat as I tried to suck it in and pose in different configurations in my bedroom — as if I could hold a fat-sucking pose all day.

When I wrote the words "put together," I felt flooded with the storied history of this phrase when it comes to women's appearances. There's no doubt that was at play here, but also, I have spent enough time full-time mothering in the last few years to know what it is to feel totally dishevelled. Society's ideals or not, it's not a lovely feeling. My sense is that I don't feel like myself in this state. Or, I should say, if I haven't been camping in the wilderness without a bathroom mirror or shampoo for days but have instead been enjoying hikes and starlit campfires, I don't feel like myself in this state.

And so, with this fairly simple experiment, I seemed to have successfully eliminated the negative feelings that can come with *not being able to find anything to wear,* or to have *nothing that fits.* I have saved myself a good deal of heartache. Another thing that I realized was quite revolutionary about this experiment is that in the past, I would often only *reward* myself with the purchase of clothing once I had earned it by losing weight. I considered buying clothing for my fatter, less ideal (in my mind) body a waste of money because hopefully I would not be this fat for long, and never again, too. Some of my underlying thinking was that if I bought clothes that fit and looked good on my larger body then I might never be motivated to lose weight. Clothes that fit were something I did not deserve.

Some of what surfaced in The Adornment Experiment was that there was a part of me that actually believed that no one else could see how fat I am but me. Unless I said it, unless I talked about it or drew attention to it, I hoped no one would see me as a fat person. This was a deeply engrained part of the denial story that I carried about my weight through my entire life. It is the luxury, perhaps, I might have had as someone who's never been *extremely* overweight; I have always carried what society would define as an "extra" thirty pounds or so, no more, and often less. An instrumental part of keeping that information to myself has been the practice of draping myself in pretty clothing that eludes the eye, and allows me to showcase the parts of me that I think are quite lovely and hide the parts of me that I find too large.

The most challenging part of getting to this point — post-baby-number-two and as heavy as I've ever been — is that I no longer felt like I could hide my size very well at all anymore. My sense was, increasingly, that people would see me as a Fat Person. That they would slot me into the Fat category (and everything I imagined came with it, including: unable, in-active, slow, unadventurous, unattractive, unhealthy).

This experience wasn't so much about being concerned about what people think, but rather feeling as though the person I was presenting to the world — my physical shape — was different than the person I was in-side. My sense of dissonance was deep and pervading.

As a new business owner at this time in my life, I had been fully thrust into the public eye, into the experience of meeting a lot of new people a lot of the time. Before this, I was at least able to have some confidence that the majority of my friends and acquaintances saw me as someone who was, indeed, able, active, fast and adventurous, who had gained some weight after having had children, and who could still outpace many on a day hike and out swim the best of them. Despite my added weight, my *ability,* or even my *former ability,* helped me to hold fast to an identity I felt I could be proud of. But now, as I was meeting new people who didn't know me as a person who could *do* all these things, as a woman who had broken a marathon swimming record or who bike-commuted a hundred kilometres a week for ten years, I felt very disconnected from the part of my identity that was able to rebel against the stereo-types people had about overweight individuals. I suddenly felt like I was a *walking stereotype*, in fact, especially having actually *lost* a lot of my physical capability over the span of my child-bearing and postpartum years with my son.

I realized that being "able" made being fat more okay to me. If I thought that someone was judging me — or even just notic-ing me — for being fat, I would casually talk about my 4km swim session that morning and feel better. It felt good, but it also served to fuel my denial that I was, indeed, fat. It was me saying, *"look at all the things I can do! I can't possibly be THAT fat, can I? Maybe no one else notices!"*

The Bodyworker Experiment…and other somatic tricks

*A*nother experiment I felt called to was one of working with a number of bodyworkers and somatic experiences — some familiar to me at the time, like massage, and some less familiar, like osteopathy. I wanted two things from these experiences: a chance to connect with my body and honour it, and a chance to invite healing to my chronic overexercise— induced pain.

The experience of regularly scheduling massages, sensory deprivation floats and Reiki treatments during this experiment was lovely, and not something I was unaccustomed to. Often, in the past, however, I would use these experiences as a way to *treat* myself for being *good.* As in, your body will deserve this when you've behaved well enough (eating well and exercising, primarily) to earn it. In this experiment, the act of regularly scheduling these things – and not waiting to do so for some weight loss or clothing size milestone – actually felt quite nourishing.

Going to visit an osteopath was probably the most fascinating experience of this experiment. My osteopath's understanding of the way my body functioned was different than any I'd known before, despite having seen many bodyworkers for various injuries over the years. I was continually in awe and wonder of how she was manipulating my body and why, exactly.

"So, when you move my arm like that while pressing into my belly….does that mean that those two things are connected??"

She talked about how the fascia in my body connected the experience I had of my organs like my heart and my uterus, with my musculoskeletal experience. Also, there was something in the way she *manipulated* my body that said: *"This is no big deal. You have a body and it works like every other body."* She did a lot of work on my belly, and at first, being touched in this area felt incredibly vulnerable, as it holds most of the shame I feel about the way my body looks and feels. But she would get this far-off look in her eyes and I would see that she was just *feeling my organs.* She gave literally no fucks about the fact that there was fat there. Her expression said to me, *"yeah, and some people are fat. Whatevs."*

The other thing that was somewhat profound about this experience was that my osteopath gave me a fairly clean bill of health at the end of our first 4-5 intensive sessions together. She felt as though my body was *functioning just as it should.* I had been and still do experience a lot of pain that comes as a result of my years of overexercising and I have had healer after bodyworker after medical provider pathologize me and my body over and over again. I hadn't realized that I had had unwittingly adopted such a schema of *brokenness* until all of a sudden I had the experience of someone *not* seeing me that way. I was living with the remnants of an unhealthy "healthy" lifestyle, but functioning fairly optimally regardless. This notion of "healthiness" would continue to be a thread that I would pick up on throughout my experimentation, and I was surprised to realize how *unhealthy* and *broken* I assumed I was.

The Meal Planning Experiment

In this experiment, I had finally decided that I had enough of a foundation in self-nourishment that I was ready to start narrowing in on the more triggering and challenging of the experiments in my body acceptance journey. At this point in my process, following the same logic I had always followed when it came to my body, I believed that changes to my food and exercise were where acceptance would *truly* lie, at the heart of it all. Unlike in the past, though, this experiment wasn't about portion control or calorie counting, but rather simply making a plan to make and eat the foods that would make me feel good and that would be nourishing to my family, so that I wouldn't have to *think so hard* about what a weekly menu might look like (and, perhaps, decide I had no time or energy for this shit and order out).

As a busy working mom of two who is also a raging foodie, I have been meal planning for quite some time. My meal planning process, though, mostly consisted of browsing my saved Pinterest pins and the bookmarks in my many cookbooks for what looked enticing, and just making those things. I decided that I could cut quite a bit of work out of the "effort" of experimenting with a gentle approach to my nutrition by having a really enticing list of possibilities to choose from on any given week. I spent several hours poring through my Pins and cookbooks, pulling out the most delicious looking but also nutritionally-balanced recipes. I added some of my own ideas, and made a detailed, colour-coded, meal-coded "cheat sheet" of ideas for healthy breakfasts, snacks, lunches and dinners. I was sure to include lots of enticing vegetable options, and ideas for food that truly seemed exciting.

When I had done this in the past, my menu looked more like a wan, not-very-creative list of Good Girl Foods from a fashion magazine. You know, the "half a plate of steamed vegetables, half a baked sweet potato and a deck-of-cards-sized portion of lean protein" kind of thing. Decidedly uninspiring.

I also made sure to have options available for times when both myself and my family tended to eat foods that didn't feel good to us: there were lots of choices for quick evening meals, for comfort food and desserts, and for times when we truly didn't feel like cooking.

I noticed a few things as a result of this change. Just planning to have something like homemade pizza on a Friday night made us excited for the prospect, and that much more likely to be more enthused by cooking than by phoning in our evening's nourishment. I also noticed that I really, really love vegetables. I mean, I think I always kind of have, but with carbohydrate- loving children and a meat-loving husband, our meals often reflected their preferences, as well as my preference for making something simple that everyone will eat. I got really, really excited about the healthier options on my menu of ideas. They were more than just steamed vegetables or mashed potatoes: they were fascinating salads with proteins and nuts; they were roasted and drizzled, dressed and spiced, definitely cheesed, and combined in imaginative ways. Having the meal plan and being *actually excited about it* made it a lot easier to just choose foods that were "real" — like grown in the ground or walking on the earth, as opposed to manufactured or ordered from the take-out place down the street. Though I was careful to notice the difference between my true sense of satisfaction and the age-old diet culture ideals that I had become so accustomed to following, these gentle supports helped me to feel well-nourished in all ways.

The Tracking Experiment

During this whole experimentation period, I had approached traditional weight loss techniques with an extremely healthy dose of skepticism. Actually, ever since my Weight Watchers loss and regain, I had done this with *all* weight loss techniques. Meal planning, to me, seemed like a simple first step that actually felt very *inviting* to me. I have always loved to plan, to think about food and make new recipes, and I get a lot of gratification out of having a lovingly and carefully planned week of nourishment available to myself and my family. It requires a bit of up-front work on the weekend as I'm inventorying our pantry, freezer and fridge and creating a grocery list, but it makes the rest of the week a lot easier. We began to waste less food, spend a little less on groceries, and eat really interesting and well-thought-through meals. It was a win-win.

So meal planning escaped my skepticism, but most other things hadn't. That was probably one of the big reasons why this journey was so different than anything I've done before: because I've done Weight Watchers, I did LA Weight Loss, I have tracked calories in and out with MyFitnessPal, I've done Tim Ferris' weird Four Hour Body diet, I've eaten paleo, "clean," grain-free, carb-free, sugar-free, dairy-free and vegan.

The only clear next experiment that I could decipher at this point was to begin to track my food intake and my exercise output. Though this practice harkened back to the many weight loss methods that had failed me before, my experience with tracking in the past was that it was also fairly revelatory. I had realized, upon doing this kind of thing before, that I repeatedly drank more fancy caramel-y coffee drinks than I thought I did, and moved far less in the run of a day than I thought I did. So I bought a Fitbit, and I started doing some food diarizing. I hoped that this might be a sort of reality check — a way to better understand my body, what felt good in it, and what it needed. After so many years of dieting and overexercise, I felt like I was starting at ground zero when it came to noticing my body's actual needs.

The Fitbit brought the first revelation. My fixation on exercise as an immense physical endeavour that often involved many hours in a pool or the kind of bike excursion that required me to let someone know where I would be and when to go driving around looking to scrape me up off the side of the road was alleviated somewhat. I realized that I was averaging around 4000-5000 steps in the run of a fairly sedentary day. And so I *simply began to walk more,* to see how it felt. Where I had convinced myself before that I didn't have enough time (particularly for the kind of exercise I had come to value), I suddenly *found* time. I bounded up the stairs to fetch *yet another* forgotten thing from my kids' bedrooms with gratitude. I walked to work more often. Even just one lap around the cul-de-sac in my neighbourhood would count for something.

And here's the thing: I had a strongly defined schema of what "worthy" exercise was in my mind – the long swims and epic bike rides – and most *certainly not* the mere act of walking. But as I began this project, I realized that although I identified as a person who did exercise in the extreme, my grandiose conceptualizations of what valuable time spent moving my body looked like had actually prevented me from doing *anything at all.* I began to feel healthier and stronger, just by walking more. I lost the ego around exercise: at the very least, even on days that I couldn't swim or ride or hit up a yoga class, I could walk.

Tracking my food intake was an entirely different challenge, however, which I ended up pursuing and giving up multiple times before I felt that I could do it in a meaningful, untriggering, and sustainable way. I tried to make it as easy as possible for myself, with apps and reminders, and I would inevitably end up forgetting to write down my intake and the whole thing would go out the window. I think, subconsciously, the whole thing felt a little bit like punishment:

12 almonds.
1 cup of tea, 1 teaspoon sugar and 1 tablespoon milk

Dammit!! Why didn't I have 10 almonds? And look at that sugar in my tea again. Really need to cut that out. Maybe switch to coconut sugar?

When I finally found a method of food diarizing I could stick to, I chose not to write in quantities unless they were notable — i.e.: more or less than usual. I gave myself a finite timeframe to track for, so that the whole thing didn't feel like *this new thing I was now going to do for the rest of my life to try to control my eating,* which felt all too diet-y to me. And I tracked EVERYTHING. I mean everything, even my poops, with a little brown pen and some cryptic symbols, lest anyone get a hold of my food diary somehow and, in doing so, obtain a detailed record of my regularity. Probably most importantly, I tracked how I felt before and after meals. I tracked how hungry

I was before and after meals. I wrote down why I decided to eat what I ate, and how satisfying it was. I jotted in the margins, in red, what my energy levels were like. I made a note of when I felt unwell, or sluggish. I wrote down when I meditated, and how many hours of sleep I got on any given night.

My goal was to not only observe my eating patterns, but also the way I felt when I ate the foods I chose, both physically and emotionally, as a way of becoming more mindful of my relationship with food, inside and out.

Through my tracking experiment, I noticed a good many things that were profound in their ordinariness. My energy levels were nearly always great. I drank lots of water, and had walked my way out of the "sedentary lifestyle" category on my FitBit. I managed to get about seven hours of sleep per night.

I also found tendencies and habits that, although they were quite "usual" for me, when written on a piece of paper, made me see them more starkly, in a way that I could more deeply consider than I had before. I had a tendency to let myself get too hungry. I would get caught up in my work, or, in the mornings especially, I would be so uncertain of what I wanted to eat that I would go hungry instead of eating something that was *not quite right*. Caffeine made me very uncomfortable. When I drank coffee, my heart would pound and I would feel nervous and flighty. I found I had some habits — not intuitions but straight-up habits — about eating desserts and sweets. I craved dessert after lunch but not necessarily dinner. I often ate sweets out of compulsion, but not necessarily hunger or even a deep desire. I got a ridiculous amount of enjoyment and satisfaction out of simple, home cooked meals. This seemed obvious to me, but I was surprised to find that my satisfaction with a simple meal made at home was actually higher than it was, generally, when I ate a restaurant meal that I had been craving.

The hard numbers in this experiment didn't lie. Out of the twenty-five days that I tracked my habits, I got eight days of exercise (other than walking), I grabbed a breakfast sandwich at a drive-through on nine of those days, I ate fourteen meals out (other than breakfast), and I bought my favourite fancy caramel-y coffee only five of those days (even though it felt like I was drinking it all the time). These numbers were fascinating to me because I thought of myself as an active person who cooked meals at home and didn't eat out much, who basically lived off of fancy caramel-y coffee. Noticing my *actual* habits, in this case, was quite eye-opening. I was surprised at how off my own perception of myself was! I didn't generate a lot of value-based judgement around this revelation, but it was interesting to me to notice that I behaved differently than I thought I did.

The Education Experiment: Intellectualizing My Body Love

As a sometimes painfully cerebral person, I am wont to intellectualize everything. When it comes to more corporal matters like the one at hand, that can be to my detriment, finding me overanalyzing my consumption habits and reasons for eating and for engaging in every manner of self-destructive behaviour. This has always usually been at the expense of actually doing anything about the issue.

But for my deep dive into the exploration of my own body love and acceptance, I really wanted to hear from thought-leaders and evidence-makers on the subject, but in a way I hadn't engaged with before. I had no interest in reading another diet book: I wanted objective, scientific evidence.

I had endeavoured to track my exercise and eating habits to bring some mindfulness and awareness to those aspects of my life, and to hopefully start to notice what *felt good in my body,* what felt like *me again.* But as I endeavoured to do this, I also realized through this experimentation that I had *no time,* anymore, for anyone else telling me that finding peace and comfort within my own skin could simply be done by eating healthy food and moving my body more. Aside from any of the obvious oversights that that perspective takes (metabolism, anyone?), while that approach may be true for many, the "not-so-simple" part is that food and movement and the way I have felt in my own skin have been areas of my life that I have always had deeply complex relationships with. I have spent many, many years associating food with both comfort and shame, nourishment and guilt, and the decision to eat less or eat better has always come laden with a motherlode of stories and beliefs and values that refuse to be swayed by the skinny-happy-be-like-me perpetuator of the latest diet craze. And I know that my relationship with exercise has been deeply problematic and in fact injurious to me in the past.

And so I sought out some different perspectives.

I started, fairly randomly, with the book *Face Value: The Hidden Ways Beauty Shapes Women's Lives*. In it, author Autumn Whitefield-Madrano presents refreshingly nuanced thoughts about beauty. Not necessarily solely regarding beauty-of-body, per se, this book explores the science behind beauty as well as the bad rap that the quest for beauty gets in our society. We're quick to blame the media for presenting unrealistic images of women. I know I've often shunned the whole idea of beauty altogether — which has resulted in me essentially "not trying." I'm a no-makeup kind of gal, and I don't think twice if the clothes I leave the house in have the remnants of my children's breakfast on them. I don't really think about whether or not others find me beautiful, and though I appreciate feeling beautiful when I do, it's not something I strive for. *Face Value* helped me to see beauty as something that actually *does* have some inherent value, and I started thinking about my own beauty (*it even feels weird to write that…"my own beauty"*) a little bit more. The book made me want to do a few beauty experiments: I wore mascara a couple times. It made my eyes pop; I liked it. I bought a red lip stain, and I felt pretty good wearing that, too. I noticed how I felt when I adorned myself with beautiful scarves or jewellery — one of my favourite things to do. How great it feels to have a lovely new hair cut and colour. I realized that I equate the quest for beauty with *frivolousness*. I assign little to no value to beautification — it has always seemed to me like a waste of time — time that I would rather spend standing in the hot shower a few minutes longer, or lingering over my morning tea. And yet spending a few minutes just to look nice made me feel good.

And, I can't help but remind myself, my lifelong obsession with the way my body looked and felt took up a lot more of my precious time than most people's morning beauty routine.

These tiny acts — swiping on some lip colour and throwing on a scarf — weren't exactly the kinds of things I pictured myself doing on this journey toward body acceptance. My previous attempts at fostering self-love and acceptance have involved "the obvious" — food and exercise. But inherent in my decision to wear makeup occasionally and adorn myself is a sense of self-worth. That I am worthy of beauty *even though I am fat.* Even when I am fat.

For me, "treating myself" to these kinds of acts of beautification was always something that was tied to some weight-loss or personal transformation accomplishment. And so it is meaningful that I have been able to offer myself a few very basic acts of personal care *without strings attached.* Without having to *be good* first.

I couldn't engage in thinking about my physical body without seeking the words and wisdom of my grandmother-by-choice (if only she knew!), Clarissa Pinkola Estes. Dr. Estes, most famously known as the author of "*Women Who Run With The Wolves,*" is a storyteller, wise woman and surrogate grandmother figure to so many women who are learning to access their own power as wise women. I see Dr. Estes as the figurehead of the rising feminine in our culture. She created an audiobook called *The Joyous Body*, and in it, she talks about our bodies as "consorts." I was fascinated by the image she conjured of our bodies as loyal consorts who just keep on functioning, heart beating, brain thinking, and otherwise generally *working*, despite the way we treat them and talk about them, punish them and try to make them fit into the mould of the "perfect body" created by our culture.

I was encouraged to read *"Women, Food and God"* by Geneen Roth, by many. This book really helped me to uncover what, exactly, might be the underlying mental and emotional processes and triggers beneath my eating habits. Roth talks about how food is inherently linked to our emotions (of course), and what it might mean to eat mindfully. In the book, Roth says,

"Unmet feelings obscure our ability to know ourselves. As long as we take ourselves to be the child who was hurt by the unconscious parent, we will never grow up. We will never know who we actually are. We will keep looking for the parent who never showed up, and forget the one who is no longer a child."

This deeply resonated with me, as I've been engaged in literature — and the act — of conscious, empathetic, attachment-style parenting with my children. I can see the hurt that my compulsive and unconscious parenting can wreak upon my own children. And, in exploring my upbringing and personal history around food, eating and my body, I know that there are aspects of my eating habits, specifically, that could be linked to deeply-held childhood narratives about emotional safety and self-worth.

Another gem from this book was the ability to recognize myself as a permissive eater rather than a restrictive eater. Restrictive eaters, as you can imagine, are people who get their kicks by restricting their eating and dieting, counting calories, and creating lots of rules around eating. They are, as Roth describes, fearful of chaos. Permissive eaters tend to have an "aw fuck it" attitude that I recognize well. When I am on a diet, it is usually never long (sometimes a week; the longest I've made it was 6 months) before I start to want to rebel against the rules. "Rules are dumb!" my hungry little self will declare. And more realistically, I just cannot fully get behind the idea of eating according to "rules" for any extended period of my life. I just can't go there. Eventually, you have to eat like a normal human being again, and you have to rely on YOURSELF, not the rules, to do that in a way that feels good. So why not cut to the chase?

My problem with this perspective has always been that I manage to generate rules for myself regardless of not believing in them. You see, I have always *made* rules really well, but I don't follow them well at all. So my new rule might be "eat more vegetables. See if you can have vegetables with every meal," or "drink a glass of water before deciding if you're really hungry," or "have protein, fat, and carbohydrates with every snack." This all sounds very reasonable, until my mind recognizes these as rules. You might think *why would you rebel against vegetables, or water?* You *like* vegetables and water! Doesn't matter. My mind wants to rebel. It is in my nature. Turns out, it's in *everyone's* nature, and it's one of the main contributors to our inability to stick to restrictive eating of any kind for a long duration of time.

In *Women, Food and God,* Roth advises that permitters need to extend the duration of time between the impulse to eat and the action of eating. To me, this was all well and good, except if you say *"Maltesers,"* I might actually be thinking about picking up a bag of those crunchy little dreamballs for three days before I finally tear into one. My dialogue will then be, *"I waited THREE days for these little buggers! Now I REALLY deserve them."*

But Roth has a few other great suggestions, too. She advises that permitters really need to learn to recognize cues for hunger, *and they need to recognize that they have a body.* She says that where restricters will often deny what their mind is thinking in favour of reducing the size of their body, permitters will deny that their body has needs in favour of satisfying cravings that are solely of the *mind.* Roth says that permitters might ask themselves the following questions:

"Were you hungry when you chose your food?"
"If you weren't physically hungry, was there another kind of hunger present?"
"Did your food taste like you thought it would taste?"
"Did it do what you thought it would do?"

This started to resonate with me more deeply: the idea that I may experience both physical hunger and emotional hunger. After reading this book, I became more aware of how I was feeling when I chose to eat food — especially food that is usually linked, for me, with a compulsion of some kind. The

Maltesers. The late-night peanut butter cookies (you know the kind — the ones you can whip up with just a cup of peanut butter, an egg and half a cup of sugar? The ones that offer literally *no barrier* to the consumption of sweets, despite one's careful attempt to have no sweets in the house….it has yet to occur to me not to buy the *peanut butter*).

The next book I picked up along my journey of understanding food and weight was *Intuitive Eating,* by Evelyn Tribole and Elyse Resch. This book seemed to me like an extension of what Roth talked about in *Women, Food and God* — that idea of acknowledging both mind and body when it came to eating, that your body may well crave very different foods than your mind does, and that insofar as what your mind craves, what it might *really* be doing is using food to satisfy a craving of another kind altogether. Food is just the *easy* way to satisfy that craving rather than, say, having a difficult conversation, feeling grief, or overcoming a childhood trauma.

As much as I began to totally embrace the premise behind intuitive eating, this book *still* got a little too rulesy for me, and it also didn't dive into the complexity of a person's psychological need for nourishment as much as I noticed in *Women, Food and God.* To me, the core of intuitive eating, distilled down to a mere concept, was about inviting some more mindfulness to the process of choosing and eating foods, and then noticing what impact those foods have on the body. The authors offered some suggestions on food alternatives for the times when what you're really craving is comfort, or self-nourishment, but they were more along the lines of "take a nice bath" than "figure out how your mother's lifetime of dieting impacted your way of thinking about food" or "unravel the complexities of living in a world that tells you over and over again that you should be a size two." But all this was still important food for thought.

A friend reminded me of the viral video by documentary filmmaker Taryn Brumfitt that had circulated around the internet a year or more ago: the one based on her experience of being a mom of three kids who decided to "get her body back" by training for a bodybuilding competition, and then, deciding that wasn't the kind of life or body she wanted to or could sustain, returned to a fairly average, healthy size. She posted a picture of the latter as an "after" picture, and of her bodybuilder's frame as the "before," and the mindfuck that caused on the internet — the *possibility* that a woman could be more satisfied with a larger, curvier, softer body — was spectacular. The viral video was a Kickstarter for a documentary that Brumfitt went on to make called *Embrace*. When the documentary finally came out, I decided to get a group of my women friends together to watch it.

One of the first things I noticed as I watched the documentary was my somewhat cynical attitude toward Brumfitt. Brumfitt talks about the origins of creating *Embrace,* sharing that she had always struggled with her body image and that after having three children she felt worse about herself than she ever had. She decided to begin bodybuilding training and describes it as *"the most gruelling sixteen weeks of my life."* She then says that after the event she was training for was over she decided she didn't like the way this new lifestyle made her feel, and so she "went back to just eating healthy and gained a bit of weight back and haven't been so confident in my body since" (essentially). Something inside me wanted to call out "bullshit!" Sixteen weeks? And then she just started eating healthfully and BOOM? That was it? This backstory, which happened at the beginning of the documentary, made me question Brumfitt's "credibility," in a way. The problem was that the "what it takes" to be healthy and accept your body was grossly oversimplified in the documentary, and *my* problem was that I noticed myself thinking *how could she possibly understand me, or all the other fat women out there, without a long and storied history of body hatred, weight loss and regain? How could SHE be the face and body behind this documentary — a beautiful, confident, white-skinned, blonde-haired woman who was really only ever-so-slightly soft around the edges?* This part of me was convinced that if a *really* fat person who had truly had a lifelong struggle with obesity made this documentary, it might look and sound a little different.

Feeling this way was fascinating to me: this may or may not have been a valid point, but it was a viscerally real reaction for me as I was watching the film. I noticed that I was denying other women their struggles with their weight based on my judgment of the body I saw them in. To me, anyone even remotely smaller than me was lucky to look the way they did and therefore couldn't possibly have "body issues." Anyone my size or larger was allowed to hate their bodies. The documentary clearly demonstrated otherwise in many ways, not the least of which was the sheer number of healthy-looking women who reported hating their bodies, to the point of experiencing body dysmorphia and disordered eating.

Another big revelation for me during this documentary was one that I've known about for a long time, but that I *heard* differently this time around. This revelation was around the tremendous influence that our culture has on how we value our bodies, and the conspiracy afoot to cause people to hate themselves and therefore spend oodles of money on diets, clothes, supplements and other products in order to achieve a body image that more closely matches the ones that are being marketed to us.

I have known about this for a long time: I have seen the Photoshop time lapse videos that show how dramatically a woman can be altered to look "beautiful" in the eyes of our thin-worshipping public. I am aware of all the airbrushing. But getting older and becoming more critical of what I see in front of me, and realizing the deeply problematic marketing ploys that are used to affect companies' bottom line by manipulating the general public, made me see this in a different way. I can see that there are a lot of people making a shit-ton of money by making me feel crappy about my body. They're even making a shit-ton of money making *men* think that women's bodies should look a certain way, thus contributing indirectly — or perhaps even *more* directly — to (hetero) women's dissatisfaction with their appearance. I started to more meaningfully question my ideas around what was a "valuable" or "desirable" body shape, as well as what was considered *healthy*.

I've long adored the term "fit fat," and used it to describe the status of my body and physical ability on many occasions. I have spent the large majority of my adult years in this category: I was bigger than many of my peers, but I could out-run, out-swim, out-bike or out-hike them any day of the week. And yet it still felt a bit revelatory for me that it might be possible for *health* to be the ONLY potentially valid way to assess or measure up a person's body, rather than by all the other markers and measures we have been taught have value[1].

Yet still, at the end of the *Embrace* documentary, as we sat in my living room, my question to my peers remained rooted in this concept that thinness equals health. I said, *"How do I balance this concept of loving and accepting my body against the fact that there is a worldwide obesity epidemic?"*[2]

What I see now that I couldn't see then, inherent in that statement, was this:

1) People who are fat shouldn't love their bodies because if they do, then they won't have the desire to get healthier, they'll become complacent and will remain fat...

2)....and fat is unhealthy.

3)....and that the *real* problem here is a *HEALTH* problem. (because, I think, that's what we default to as the socially acceptable reason for wanting to change our fat bodies or wanting others to change their fat bodies. It's not cool to say that fat people are ugly or less-valued members of society, so we just say they're UNHEALTHY)

4) ...the concept behind the action or decision to love one's body is deeply conflated with feeding it healthy food and

---

[1] Even the value we, as a society, place on health, is controversial. Many fat activists argue that health and healthiness – challenging to define as they are – are values that not everyone shares, and that we, as individuals, don't owe anyone our health if that is not a value we ourselves uphold.

[2] Remember that this is written in *almost* real-time, and this statement reflected my thinking at the time. In fact, the "obesity epidemic" has been contested by many - keep reading to find out more about the scientific evidence behind what is known as "the obesity paradox."

exercising, which quickly becomes enmeshed in the Diet Culture

5) That Culture tells me that the only valuable bodies are thin bodies, that healthy equates to thin….and here are 154,586 products that you can buy to make yourself thin and beautiful and *healthy*.

It started to dawn on me that the world — and I — lack a schematic by which a fat person could be healthy. We lack a schematic by which a fat person might be beautiful. We lack a schematic within which a fat person could be valued, normal, happy with themselves, could *not* want OR NEED to change their bodies. Part of me recognized that I had been so deeply acculturated to believe that fat and health could not co-exist in the same body that even as I typed this I was thinking *"of course we don't have a schematic by which fat people might be healthy, beautiful, normal and valued: there are people who can't fit through doorways and people who need cranes to lift them out of bed and people who live in pain and listlessness from consuming junk food."* Of course, though, this may be both true *and* irrelevant to the vast majority of us fat folks who feel oppressed and shamed but do not need heavy machinery to allow us to participate in the activities of daily living.

And we can't deny that even as there are people making boat-loads of money telling us we're too fat and trying to get us to spend money getting thin, one glance at the average city block or inside my local grocery store tells me that there are *also* a lot of people making a lot of money selling me food that is laden with sugar to instil cravings for more, that is cleverly packaged to appeal to my busy lifestyle, that is mass-produced and processed beyond belief and marketed to me ad nauseam.

All this made me unsure *what* I should trust.

It made me feel like all I could trust was myself.

But alongside this feeling came the question: if I have been so deeply engrained to believe, from the very beginning of my life, that fat is bad, certain foods are unhealthy, that eating less is good (etc…etc…etc…) — how could I even *truly* have my own thoughts and feelings about food and my body, unless I lived in a cave or something? How do I separate my acculturated beliefs from the *actual, literal* feelings of my body? I know enough about the power of my brain over my body and my perceptions to know that if I'm told something is healthy, there's a good chance that that suggestion will have a psychosomatic effect on me, causing me to notice feelings of increased health and vigour as a result. The evidence is everywhere. Take all the low-fat products that were all the rage in the 90s. We know now that many of those products were actually amped up with sugar to increase the flavour, so they were unhealthy as all hell (by our current sugar-hating standards), but they had less fat, and fat, at the time, was the devil (kind of like sugar is now). So I am sure that all of us *felt* healthy when we downed those tubs of fat-free yogurt, because we were too acculturated to believe that it *would* make us feel healthy to feel any other way. It's highly unpopular to suggest that anything within the current dietary trend might *not* feel wonderful in your body, might have no apparent health benefit, or, even, might be detrimental to your health. For example, when I asked a nutritionist friend if it might be possible that gluten-laden bread might NOT wreak total havoc on my body, she looked at me like I had three heads. How could I actually pay attention to how bread *felt* in my body with a response like that?

All this left me feeling uncertain, and tired, and it made living in a cave look *really* appealing.

Despite my overwhelm, something else happened when I watched the *Embrace* documentary. I saw a woman named Linda Bacon speak, and I was intrigued by what she said. She is the leader of a movement called HAES: Health At Every Size. The whole idea that fat might not have to equal unhealthy, and that the diet industry has led us to believe that it is not just unhealthy but unacceptable to be fat — and is making oodles and oodles of money doing so — struck a chord with me. I wanted to learn more.

A Paradigm Shift

– rebellion –

"A diet is the most ubiquitous and violent act of compliance there is, because you've been brainwashed to think that you can't trust yourself or your body. You've bought into one of body submission's main messages: you're out of control." — Rachel Cole

In the oft-cited concept of *the Heroine's Journey*, there comes a point in a woman's quest for her own truth at which she is called to shed old ways of thinking – even old ideas about her very *identity* – to make way for the new.

Spoiler alert: that's what happened next. Be warned: this is the point at which this whole book, and all the experiments in it, take a dramatic turn.

This shift in my journey surprised me just as much as it might surprise you, and I understand if you're not ready to read this, not ready to engage with it. Not everyone is; I definitely, most certainly was. This new perspective on my body, my health, and my size, was exactly what I was looking for, and began to inform an entirely new way of relating to myself.

I started out this journey of trying to find peace with my body by attempting to recreate the situations under which I had previously lost weight, but doing so in a way that felt more sane and more sustainable to me. Of course, I'm delighted to report that as a result I much more consistently hydrate my body with lots of water, my pits don't stink, I wear lovely clothing that makes me feel good most of the time, I go for regular massages and I meal plan consistently (which is enjoyable for me). Something inside me was still resistant to going down the path of actually restricting my eating in any way, but I didn't have another schema by which I could imagine finding a place of acceptance in my own skin.

Finding the work of Linda Bacon at the end of my first year of tiny experiments changed everything. More specifically, it was finding the movement she's created — Health At Every Size — that shifted my entire perspective on everything I knew about my weight, and the years I'd spent trying to get rid of it.

Health at Every Size is Bacon's first book, and it created a massive ripple effect in the world of dieticians, nutritionists, fat activists, and chronic dieters everywhere. To the fore, Bacon brought research that indicates that, first of all, diets don't work. This knowledge stems from a robust body of evidence (that is ignored by the majority of the world) that indicates though diets may work in the short term (within the first year or maybe two), fully 95% of people who diet regain the weight they lost, and often more, within five years of having originally lost it.

95%. Ninety. Five. Percent.

Oddly, rather than feeling completely hopeless about any future I might have of losing the weight I'd gained, this statistic caused me to breathe a big sigh of relief. I wasn't flawed in some way for not being able to lose weight and keep it off. It's just how bodies — almost *all* bodies, including mine — work.

The science behind it is this: when we restrict our diet significantly, both physiological and psychological factors rush in to protect us from ourselves. Physiologically, our inner cave-man sits up and says, "shit! we're starving!" and begins to slow our metabolism, burning fewer calories and causing that nasty "plateau effect" that anyone who's dieted before can attest to. Psychologically, when we are told we can't have something, WE WANT IT. Holy sweet mother of god, do we ever. Cravings are the primary complaint of dieters. While sometimes those crav-ings are physiological in origin (i.e.: people craving salt, for ex-ample, could actually be craving more or different minerals in their diet), many cravings are a part of a complex web of psy-chological influences. And the more we deny ourselves, the more we want. And so, what ends up happening to the vast ma-jority of dieters (myself included) is that they restrict and re-strict and restrict their eating, and then all of a sudden have a massive bingefest. They then punish themselves either physical-ly or psychologically, get back on the "bandwagon" and repeat the cycle ad nauseam.

I'm not just talking about what happens in *my* kitchen. There is an abundance of evidence to support this phe-nomenon. Herman, Polivy and Esses (1987) assert that com-pared to non-restrained eaters, adults who are restrained eaters tended to "counter-regulate": eating disproportionately large amounts in response to stress and to external cues like the presence of attractive food. This was the research that sparked the beginnings of our understanding of the starvation-binge cycle that so many of us, including myself, have experienced. These authors then went on to do the research that began to demonstrate that dieting actually *makes people fat*.

This diet-binge cycle can really fuck up our metabolism, especially when considered on the macro level – when we're talking not just about one night with three bags of Miss Vickie's, but an entire duration of time dieting followed by regain.

Not to mention, the languaging society gives us about "cheating" and "getting back on the bandwagon" is totally self-destructive, and even more so because it is essentially self-hatred bottled up and labelled as self-care.

This cycle is nothing less than *disordered eating*. It may or may not lead to an actual *eating disorder*. As I learned and began to fully comprehend this research, I was completely floored to see my dieting history through the lens of being *disordered*. As soon as I saw it that way, I could see how self-destructive it actually was (see also: hiding in a closet with a jar of Nutella, admonishing myself for having no will power).

It was at this time, after having my world rocked by HAES, that I remembered the work of Ellyn Satter, a Registered Dietician and therapeutic Social Worker, which my naturopath had introduced me to several years ago when I was struggling with feeding my picky kids.

Satter is a proponent of "normal eating," which she defines as follows:

"Normal eating is going to the table hungry and eating until you are satisfied. It is being able to choose food you like and eat it and truly get enough of it — not just stopping eating because you think you should. Normal eating is being able to give some thought to your food selection so you get nutritious food, but not being so wary and restrictive that you miss out on enjoyable food. Normal eating is giving yourself permission to eat sometimes because you are happy, sad or bored, or just because it feels good.

Normal eating is mostly three meals a day, or four or five, or it can be choosing to munch along the way. It is leaving some cookies on the plate because you know you can have some again tomorrow, or it is eating more now because they taste so wonderful. Normal eating is overeating at times, feeling stuffed and uncomfortable. And it can be undereating at times and wishing you had more. Normal eating is trusting your body to make up for your mistakes in eating. Normal eating takes up some of your time and attention, but keeps its place as only one important area of your life.

In short, normal eating is flexible. It varies in response to your hunger, your schedule, your proximity to food and your feelings."

Reading this definition felt different to me than the philosophy behind *Intuitive Eating,* which, along with *Health at Every Size,* is a veritable Bible in this entire subculture of outspoken activists that I felt so deeply fortunate to discover. When I had read *Intuitive Eating,* the principles of the philosophy still made it feel a bit like a diet to me. In fact, I came to realize this was a symptom of me beginning to develop a "red flag system" for Diets That Seem Like a Really Good Idea and Actually Aren't: if there are rules and ways of being that I have to *memorize* (aka look outside of my own intuitive and instincts and toward some externally-created "rule") then it makes me *highly skeptical.* And, after having immersed myself in the literature on intuitive eating and health at every size, I came to realize that there are a great many diets out there masquerading as Not-Diets. Clean eating, for example, which places a very definitive value of "cleanness," and everything that comes with it, on certain foods. The subtext is that anything you eat outside of what is considered "clean" is dirty, not allowed, shameful, and ultimately punishable by way of guilt trips and further restriction. The same thing goes for things like Whole Thirty, which seems, at first glance, like a fairly straightforward "Eat Real Food approach." And while it makes lots of sense for us to eat foods that come from the earth and not a factory, and in fact eating those foods may make many people feel really great, the problem lies within the restrictive mentality regarding "Real Foods." Placing a value or judgment around that jar of Nutella, as the research shows, makes most people just *really want Nutella* (and then eat it, and then rather than paying attention to how it tasted, or how they felt in their *actual bodies* afterwards, they focus on how crappy they feel about breaking the rules, how they have no willpower, and how they need to go for a run now).

Ellen Sattyr's definition of normal eating also allows for *emotional eating* in a way that the intuitive eating philosophy doesn't. Emotional eating gets a *really bad rap,* but here's the thing: we are taught, literally from the moment we emerge from the womb, that we can and should eat for emotional reasons. It sort of shocks me, when I really think about it, that as a doula I'm constantly telling women to remember that their baby *may* want to breastfeed for the sake of obtaining nutrients, but that it's *perfectly okay* and actually *normal* to breastfeed your baby for a whole host of other reasons: because your baby is crying and you want to comfort him, to help your baby go to sleep, or when you just want to connect with your baby.

(This approach consistently and unsurprisingly gets frowned upon by many grandmothers and mothers-in-laws, and I'm starting to realize that that disdain comes not just as a product of a world that didn't understand the fundamentals of safe and secure infant attachment in the way that we do now, but also was laden with a heavy dose of Diet Culture)

One of the other activists I discovered down this rabbit hole of *Health at Every Size*, Isabel Foxen Duke, has this to say about emotional eating:

> *"Eating IS emotional. Food, like sex, has an impact on the way we feel. The effects may be temporary, but they still exist, and you're ALLOWED to utilize food as a coping mechanism if you so choose. And I know what you're thinking...'But where do I draw the line? If I let myself eat emotionally I'd NEVER STOP.' And the answer is 'YOU get to draw the line.' Wherever the hell you want to draw it. You are an adult. You can do whatever the fuck you want. Now the difference between classically-understood 'intuitive eating' and what I call 'normal eating' is that 'normal eating' merges 'intuitive eating' with a healthy dose of 'you're allowed to eat emotionally if you damn well want to. We are never going to 'eat according to our bodies' needs exclusively 100% of the time. A more realistic goal is some flexible and unprescribed negotiation between the needs of both. I honour the needs of my body AND mind in my choices with food — knowing that they won't always agree with one another. Sometimes a little compromise is in order."*

The Evidence

Everything I read about intuitive eating, normal eating, and health at every size was, on a moment by moment basis (usually corresponding to every time I made a food choice or noticed I was hungry) blowing. my. damn. mind.

But I am a researcher at heart, with a science degree, and a hefty dose of skepticism. Also, I had been conditioned, like possibly *everyone else on the planet,* to believe wholeheartedly Diet Culture's firm assertion that if only I could eat and exercise like a Good Girl, I would lose weight (and be popular....right?). Not to mention, all of this new information and this new perspective essentially meant that I had spent my entire life with a *daily* focus on my dissatisfaction with my body, and what I would do to resolve it, and all for completely, utterly, totally *naught*. I both wanted what I was learning to be true, and didn't, at the same time.

And so I went in search of The Evidence. I knew that if I were to adopt this new perspective on my body and health, that I would have to adopt it for life. This wasn't another fad, this was a total and utter paradigm shift for me, and I couldn't afford to turn back. Consequently, I couldn't afford to be wrong about this, either. I wanted research. I wanted double-blind peer-reviewed scientific studies. I wanted *proof* that diets didn't work, and that I could trust my body.

I began to get more curious about the intuitive eating approach I had learned about. I wondered: *what if I start eating intuitively and then somehow intuitively eat my way through a jar of Nutella, and NEVER STOP?* As it turns out, there are dozens of studies comparing intuitive eating, or a "non-diet" approach, with dieting. One of the most comprehensive studies I found was a literature review published in 2014 by VanDyke and Drinkwater, which found that "intuitive eating is negatively associated with BMI, positively associated with various psychological health indicators, and possibly positively associated with improved dietary intake and/or eating behaviours...The implementation of intuitive eating results in weight maintenance but perhaps not weight loss, improved psychological health, possibly improved physical health indicators other than BMI (e.g. blood pressure; cholesterol levels) and dietary intake and/

or eating behaviours." This same study found evidence that, of the research studies reviewed, the ones that included long-term follow up (this is so important because remember: the evidence shows that for many, diets assure weight loss within the first year or two, but almost always result in regain), intuitive eating helps people develop a healthier relationship with food resulting in improvements in blood pressure, lipids, and cardiorespiratory fitness — even in the absence of weight loss. In addition, intuitive eating has positive psychological benefits including decreased depression and anxiety, increased self-esteem, and improved body image.

The next big question I had was: *what about health?* Does the idea of "health at every size" really hold water when held up to the analytical scrutiny of a peer-reviewed study? Many people, including me, justify a desire to lose weight with the noble goal of improving health. That, for many of us, is the true bottom line. We say things like "I want to be around to meet my grandchildren" and other such wholesome wishes. Adopting a non-diet mentality is terrifying, for many, because we have been so engendered to believe that thin equals healthy, and so the possibility that this approach may not lead to weight loss invokes our fear of our own mortality.

As with the intuitive eating or non-diet approach to food, the evidence around health at every size — *the idea that our actual physiological indicators of health might be in the range of normal regardless of our physical mass* — is aplenty.

In a study by Linda Bacon and colleagues (2005), after a six-month intervention comparing individuals who had been offered a health at every size program or a diet program, the health at every size group maintained weight, improved in measures of metabolic fitness (blood pressure and blood lipids), eating behaviour, and psychological measures (self-esteem, body image, depression). The diet group participants lost weight and showed initial improvement in many variables, but at one year post-intervention, their weight was regained and few of the physiological and psychological improvements had been sustained.

A statement paper in the *Journal of Social Issues* by Ernsberger and Koletsky (2000) couldn't have summed up the problem with dieting as a rationale for health improvement more powerfully:

"Despite considerable moderating evidence, the prevailing wisdom is that obesity is a severely life-threatening condition. Health professionals, the media and the general public remain convinced that even modest elevations in BMI drastically shorten life expectancy and increase incidence of degenerative diseases such as heart disease, cancer and diabetes. There is abundant evidence that current thinking on extreme health risks associated with obesity has survived due to biased thinking and selective perception of both clinical practice and the literature. Obesity experts have maintained their certainty by reviewing and citing articles that assign a high risk to obesity, including relying primarily on cross-sectional morbidity studies. Obesity experts cite with far less frequency clinically unbiased mortality studies which show elevated body weight to be more benign and even show low body weight and/or weight loss to carry health risks. The resulting conviction that obesity is medically extremely dangerous has produced health policy that consistently recommends weight loss as the first line of intervention, even though it is abundantly clear that there is no method for achieving and maintaining weight loss."

This perspective, particularly as it relates to obesity management as a health intervention and as public health policy, was highlighted in further depth by Bombak in a 2014 commentary in the *American Journal of Public Health*. In this article, Bombak reminds readers that in 1992, the American National Institutes of Health (NIH) released a consensus statement that dieting is an ineffective method to produce sustained weight loss.

(Did your jaw just drop here too? Did you, like I did, start wondering how physicians and dieticians who promote weight loss can sleep at night knowing they're prescribing interventions on a daily basis that not only don't work but that are very likely to be actively harmful?)

Bombak goes on to summarize other key evidence in the argument for non-dieting and health at every size. Echoing the post-diet experience that myself and so many others have had, Bombak states "recent evidence on the physiological changes that follow weight loss in obese animal models and humans suggests organisms' endocrine systems actively promote weight regain. Such changes involve…reduced satiety, increased hunger, suppressed energy expenditure, a decrease in nutrient availability, enhanced metabolic flexibility, an increase in energy efficiency and storage in peripheral tissues, a decline in adipose energy depletion signalling from leptin and insulin, altered neural activity, and alterations in hepatic, adipose tissue and skeletal muscle metabolism. Importantly, similar changes have been identified in humans for a full year after weight loss. Such processes may help explain the very high rates of recidivism in weight-loss dieters. Given these rates of recidivism, it is concerning that weight regain is largely composed of fat. Furthermore, weight loss may not be harmless and may increase stress, release of persistent organic pollutants, and risk of osteoporosis."

If that weren't eye-opening enough, Bombak continues: "despite its widespread adoption, BMI is acknowledged to be a crude measurement of obesity…[in fact] overweight status (BMI = 25-30) has been shown to be associated with decreased mortality risk in US, Canadian and international samples. Obesity (BMI>30) has even demonstrated a protective or neutral effect among some chronic disease or older populations."

What Bombak is talking about is something increasingly known as the "obesity paradox." The paradox is that the evidence – the real, live, actual evidence around health vis-a-vis obesity – contradicts what we as a society have come to believe about obesity. Studies have shown that obese individuals with cardiovascular disease are more likely to survive than "normal weight" individuals with cardiovascular disease (Bombak 2014). In addition, a great proportion of overweight and obese individuals are metabolically healthy, and that being physically fit, even when obese, may eliminate the association between obesity and increased mortality.

The bottom line here is that health at every size is a *thing*. Despite what we as a culture have been told, it's been well-documented that weight is not a good indicator of health. Cardiovascular fitness is far more important as it has a direct effect on key indicators of decreased mortality rates, and while eating healthy foods and honouring hunger and satiety cues is key to a positive relationship with food, that relationship can easily become disordered when it is controlled to the extent it often is when we are "treated" for overweight and obesity as a method of purportedly increasing health.

Finding Role Models: The Anti-Diet Sub-Culture

"The diet industry is predicated on one idea that persists against all logic and reason even though it is a multibillion-dollar industry whose products fail the vast majority of the time. The problem isn't them — it's you. This is a system whose business plan is keeping all of us in shame as long as possible — hopefully our whole lives. And shame thrives in silence, which means we continue to blame ourselves for what in reality is a broken system that not only benefits from but actually requires our failure in order to ensure repeat customers. And why wouldn't we? Going on yet another diet, cooking up new ways to control our bodies, and putting ourselves down aren't signs of a different kind of failure in how we relate to ourselves; they're the natural response to a culture that tells us we won't be acceptable unless we do. We haven't failed. We've been failed. And now we get to do something about it."

—Anna Guest-Jelley, *Curvy Yoga*

Falling down the rabbit hole of the work of the researchers, thought-leaders and activists behind the Health at Every Size movement was probably the best thing that's ever happened to me and my sweet, misunderstood, oft-loathed body. In this anti-diet sub-culture, I was deeply inspired by women who are radically changing the way we think about bodies by defying the norms established by Diet Culture.

Many of these women also speak to the ways in which Diet Culture reinforces damaging patriarchal belief systems about women's bodies, and women's rights.

Cheryl Strayed couldn't have said it better:

"What is on the other side of the tiny gigantic revolution in which I move from loathing to loving my own skin? What fruits would that particular liberation bear? We don't know — as a culture, as a gender, as individuals, you and I. The fact that we don't know is feminism's one true failure. We claimed the agency, we granted ourselves the authority, we gathered the accolades, but we never stopped worrying about how our asses looked in our jeans. There are a bunch of reasons for this, a whole bunch of Big Sexist Things We Can Rightfully Blame. But ultimately, like anything, the change is up to us."

Part of the work that I began to do to shift my mindset when it came to my body and my health, after having discovered Health at Every Size, was to reorient the content of my inbox and my social media feeds with the wise words and images of the women who are at the forefront of this massive perspective overhaul. Seeing more curvy bodies and fewer newly-minted pyramid scheme-style weight loss coaches in my day-to-day media consumption has been deeply healing. It's hard to express what it feels like to actually recognize the bodies, and, inherently, the *lived experiences,* of the people I allow into my life and my inbox.

The result, for me, has been a sense of community and belonging to a group of people who live with similar physical experiences to me, and who also walk in a world that can make it difficult to be different, to be in a larger body. That loneliness

I always felt about being larger than my friends and therefore unable to navigate the world in the same way they did? It has started to dissipate.

Soooo…..am I actually HEALTHY???

After having my worldview *rocked* by everything I was learning about Health at Every Size and Diet Culture, I began to feel uncertain again. My sense is that a part of my identity was subtly shifting: I was navigating what it would be like to claim my fatness *and* my health *and* my worthiness in a way that I had never done before. It felt like I was trying a new sense of self on for (literal) size, and I was still afraid to step fully into what this might mean for me. It was as though I wanted to know that it was safe to try to accept my body *just as it was*.

Though I was totally *down* with the idea of intuitive and normal eating, with pleasurable, desire-based movement, with the health at every size perspective, and with beginning to trust myself to know what I needed, the woman in me who's spent the last thirty years obsessed with food and exercise still needed to know *just one more thing* before I could step fully into this new way of being and thinking.

Am I actually healthy?

What is "healthy," anyway?

I wanted to know *for certain* that I could fully embrace — and trust — a health at every size mentality, and that meant knowing that I was actually *healthy*.

Nevermind that I was a bit stymied by what I might do if I *weren't* healthy, because attempting to lose weight was officially off my bucket list now that I knew that any attempt I made would likely be met with initial success, but ultimate failure, which would leave me in a worse-off place than I was, with more muscle loss and more fat gain, with my metabolism shocked even more deeply into thinking I was starving, and with a binge response to deprivation that I didn't want to put myself through. Not to mention that a great deal of the evidence around weight being related to the health outcomes it's typically associated with was somewhat questionable when held up to higher standards of methodological rigour, as I had learned in reviewing the intuitive eating and health at every size research.

I asked around. I Googled. The naturopaths I chatted with reminded me that health is an ever-changing continuum, and so the question *"am I healthy"* was a bit difficult to pin down, unless I asked it every single minute of every single day. Also, naturopaths and Google have a very different perspective on the concept of health, a microcosm of the perspective shared by most holistic health care providers vis-a-vis their allopathic counterparts. Google reported that I could generally consider myself healthy if I had no overt physical symptoms of ailment, if my blood pressure was normal, if I had regular periods, good energy, slept well at night, and was generally happy.

As I realized that I could check the vast majority of those boxes, something else occurred to me.

I had assumed that I was *unhealthy*.

I assumed that when analyzed and measured and scanned and tested, I would be found lacking.

I believe that certainly some of this sentiment came from the messaging that I and other fat people get about the idea that fat is unhealthy (*not to mention the messaging that comes along with that which says, fat is unhealthy and unhealthy is unworthy*).

I also believe that we, as a culture, have come to have a dramatically skewed conceptualization of health. Perhaps it's modern science and the ability to understand the body better than we ever have before, or perhaps it's our deep-rooted fear of death and subsequent maniacal desire to do anything we can to prolong our lives, or perhaps it's both. Nevertheless, I would venture that the great majority of us perceive there to be *something* wrong with our bodies, our health, or ourselves. If we are lucky enough to fall into Google's and allopathic medicine's definition of health as "*the absence of disease*," then we are likely to look to other models of health and disease to pathologize ourselves. When you speak to the average person nowadays, they're apt to tell you about the many foods they're intolerant to, or that they are taking enzymes to support their liver so that they can *detoxify*. (This concept of detoxification is one that our culture is fairly obsessed with, as though we've all been slogging through a toxic waste lagoon in our spare time).

And I get it, kind of. Our environment is legitimately polluted, and the food we often consume falls more in the category of *factory-made chemical* than sustenance. We have a story of our society as being one that is more stressed out than our ancestors were (although you'll have a hard time convincing me that the possibility of being trampled by a woolly mammoth or running out of preserves during a long hard winter is less stressful than our day planners and inboxes). And there are a great many genuinely unwell people out there.

I am convinced, though, in this culture that has elevated wellness and health to the level of holiness, that we are not as ridden with pathology as we think we are.

There are a great many people making oodles of money convincing us that we are unhealthy, require detoxifying, and, in the subtext, not good enough or faulty in some way. To me, this equates to a whole lot of people who stand to profit from the assumption that our bodies don't have the wisdom and ability to regulate and process and integrate what we do to them and put in them. I think we underestimate ourselves and our bodies, and I also think that this undermines the very trust in our physiology that allows us to connect with our wellbeing enough to know when something *actually is* going on. We've come to rely on a glut of information and the expertise of others to determine where we rate on the health scale, and they're a biased lot, not poised to make a living from a society full of perfectly healthy individuals. If anything is pathological about our society, I would argue it's our persistent attempts to seek answers outside of ourselves before attuning to our own intuition first.

And so it was this perspective that I brought to the question *"am I healthy?"*

During my tracking experiment, I found that, for the most part and by most definitions of the word, I actually was healthy.

Mostly.

My primary physical ailments were the pain that I experience in my knees, the degenerative disc syndrome and subsequent pain that I experience in my lower back, and the occasional flare-up of shoulder pain, usually wrought by sleeping or nursing my son in a weird position. I know, now, after having truly recognized the extent of my overexercise in my twenties, that much of the physical pain I have now is directly related to the sheer number of injuries I sustained during that period of my life. With regular bodywork and yoga, I have come to a place where these ailments are mostly under control, where I don't experience debilitating pain with them, at least most of the time.

Right now, and for the most part, I am healthy. I am not broken. And I can listen to my own intuition about how I'm feeling, rather than ascribing to the "pathology of the day."

How Far I've *Already* Come

"I temporarily inhabit an amazing animal that is willing to suffer so that I can learn from my mistakes." — Martha Beck

Realizing my food preferences, and that perhaps my body and my intuition have been more evident in my relationship with food than I had previously thought, I started wondering: how far have I *already* come in my journey with accepting and respecting my body, and releasing the hold that Diet Culture and years of conditioning have had on me?

I think one of the first things that I did to release myself from my lifelong history of trying to "fix" my body was to stop running. During my twenties, the large majority of which I spent overexercising and dieting, I was quite obsessive about running. Although there was only a period of about a year that I can actually recall truly *enjoying* running, it remained a staple in my pursuit of thinness, ability, health and self-acceptance for nearly a decade. My obsession with it was rooted in what I imagine many people's running obsessions are: it was the most efficient calorie-burning exercise I could do. I may have preferred swimming, or hiking, or yoga, but those things weren't as effective at helping me lose weight (and counteracting my binging habits) as running was. Running could make everything okay again when my diet had gotten out of control. Running allowed me a sense of control, a sense that there was something I *could* do to lose weight, even when I couldn't figure out why I didn't have the "willpower" to avoid my chocolate cravings.

When I was pregnant with my daughter, I ran until I was about six months along. I even competed in a sprint-distance triathlon at three months gestation. At the six month point, though, the hormone relaxin that was flooding my body during pregnancy made my joints ache almost unbearably after a run, and one day, when I found myself still hobbling around several hours after having finished my workout, I realized I needed to take a break.

I ran sporadically throughout my postpartum period, but always found that it aggravated my knee pain quite significantly, and it felt *hard*. Yes, I was usually pushing a running stroller with a grumpy baby in it, but it was hard without the added effort of the stroller as well. I did not enjoy running, at all. For the next three years or so, I continued to hold the intention of running, and even went so far as to put it on my "to do" list most weeks, but I rarely went, sighing, and scribbling the word RUN out of my day planner when the time had come and gone to strap on my running shoes.

My last run was shortly after I had my son. I went out a couple times after he was born, determined to Lose the Baby Weight and sure that running would be the most efficient way, especially important now that I was juggling being a mother of two and running a business, to reduce the size of my body.

It hurt. For a week afterward, I had such pain in my knees that I winced climbing up and down the stairs, and could barely lower myself onto the toilet without yelping in pain.

I had, at that point, long since decided that the gym was not a place I was interested in (unless it had a yoga studio or a pool to swim in in the winter), and so I decided that I would focus my energy on other outdoor activities that I enjoyed, such as hiking, biking and paddling. I began to take the radical step of trying to do *exactly what I felt like* on any given day, rather that prescribing myself a weekly exercise schedule.

And gradually, I stopped calling it exercise at all. I moved my body. I did whatever my body wanted that day, whether it was stretching across a yoga mat or biking on my favourite winding road. I thought of myself and my relationship to movement much as I think of my dog and her daily requirement for walks. Movement felt good and cleared my mind, even if it was just walking a few loops around my neighbourhood, which never previously would have made "the cut" as far as qualifying as exercise. In short, I focused on how moving felt, and what I was craving, rather than thinking of it as a way to get thin, or even to stay healthy.

I realized that I needed to give myself more credit for truly healing my relationship to exercise, especially as someone who identifies as a former overexerciser, and as someone who had actually permanently injured herself as a result of that compulsion.

The other healing that had occurred in my life without my full recognition was around some of the hang-ups I had had about food. Although I often blame my years as a food blogger for a significant proportion of my weight gain, what I also learned during those years was a deep pleasure in the satisfaction of cooking, eating, and nourishing myself and others. During this time, I began to develop a philosophy, as a blogger and as a food-lover, that all foods were okay. That it was okay to deeply enjoy a piece of cake, rather than sneaking it and being ashamed of it. Blogging also made me more aware of what I came to know as "normal" eating: it introduced me to a *whole entire world* of people who thought nothing of eating thick slabs of homemade bread smeared with butter, or an exquisitely fragrant risotto. It made me realize that I wasn't very interested in participating in a worldview that would deny me those things, and I became more and more reluctant to engage in dieting behaviour. I realize that this reluctance was the seed from which my final rejection of Diet Culture grew, and for that I am endlessly grateful.

And so it is that despite the fact that I felt so *new* at the idea of unrestricted eating and intuitive movement, of nourishing and moving my body for pleasure, I came to realize that I had been nurturing and developing this perspective for quite a while, and that its time had come. Unlike the diets and exercise regimes of my past, this new paradigm, this new way of being in and thinking about my body, was here to stay.

So *Now* What the Fuck

"Then let's figure out how to help you make peace with your body. We've got to host a reunion. Bring back together your body, mind and spirit. Vote your body back on the island. Make you whole again."

— Glennon Doyle, *Love Warrior*

When I started this journey, writing this book and doing my tiny experiments in body respect and acceptance, I honestly have to say that as much as I wanted to magically manifest love for the physical form I currently occupy, deep down I thought the most likely path toward my acceptance and long-awaited peace with my body was going to be a result of losing weight. When I first embarked on this path, I thought that these tiny experiments were, actually, eventually going to be about more salad and swimming, because I was completely devoid of a worldview that did not involve those things.

And so with my perspective shift came my next question, which would come to inform the next year of my tiny experiments: now what the fuck do I do?

I knew I had reached a liminal space – a space of *not that* but *not yet this*. In the Heroine's Journey, it's this time of liminality that signals that a woman's *real journey* is about to begin.

I still had a long path ahead of me before I felt I could truly accept and maybe even love my body. But suddenly the map I had been using to guide my way was telling me I needed to take a totally different route.

It was hard to give up the idea of losing weight. Choosing not to engage in Diet Culture, and therefore not to always be trying to or wishing I could lose ten or twenty pounds was, and sometimes still is, incredibly difficult. It was hard not just because I had been doing it *literally* all my life, but also because it flies in the face of what our *entire* culture understands about weight, and about people who carry more of it than others. I felt infinitely more comfortable with the weight I'd put on since having my children (and with the weight I have always carried on my body) when I had a plan to get rid of it. When I talked about my weight and my feelings about my body with others, I became infinitely more acceptable to them when I shared that I was trying to get more exercise, or trying out a new eating regime.

I desperately wanted to start tuning into my hunger and fullness cues, adopting some of the intuitive eating practices while also keeping a healthy dose of Ellyn Satter's normal eating mentality at the forefront. But first, I wondered if maybe I needed to do a cleanse. A reset of some kind. You know — cut out gluten and dairy and sugar so that I could get a "baseline" for what makes my body feel good and what doesn't.

Something about this idea didn't sit right with me, but it clung to me nevertheless. I Pinned a bunch of Whole 30 recipe ideas and made a few meal plans, deciding that perhaps I would try Whole 30 for just a week, and see what happened.

Evidently this "one more diet" impulse is almost laughably common among people new to the non-diet mentality; and sure enough, here I was.

My rationale was the sheer number of "success stories" that I had been exposed to in which people say "I didn't realize how much (insert food here) bothered my body until I had cut it out." I thought, maybe in order to truly tune into and be intuitive about what I'm eating and how it makes my body feel, I needed to cut a whole bunch of things out and then add them back in. Maybe I'd never want to eat gluten again if I realized that I'd actually been living my entire life massively bloated!

By this time, I had found a local intuitive eating guru: ironically, the naturopath who had originally introduced me to Ellyn Satter's normal eating model had shifted her practice to support people with intuitive eating. She quickly became my go-to, and my inspiration, as I navigated the waters of giving up dieting. And she had the credibility my researcher brain had been seeking: she was a former dietician and naturopathic doctor who now believed that giving people meal plans was unethical. When I told her about my cleanse quandary, she said that really, such an approach would only be recommended if I had a serious condition that may be resolved by diet change, such as irritable bowel syndrome.

And what had I found when I had done my tracking experiment?

I was painfully normal. Regular poops and all.

The other thing that tugged at my intuition was that, based on all the evidence that I had read about food restriction, I had a fairly good chance — both statistically and *knowing me* — of rebounding off my cleanse with a binge. All the gluten, all the dairy, all the sugar. In addition, the evidence, and my history, showed that if I lost weight while cleansing, I stood a good chance of regaining it all and then some. I realized that by doing this, I would end up back at square one all over again. I had come so far in my revelations around dieting at this point, I couldn't bear the thought of turning back.

And so I made a conscious decision: I would no longer diet. No cleanses.

But at the root of that decision was something else: if I *did* have some kind of an adverse reaction to a particular food, I was going to have to listen to my body very carefully, to make sure I wasn't going to be one of those people that were somehow completely ignorant of the fact that they were intolerant to something.

And at the deepest, deepest heart of all this was *self-trust.*

Something told me that this experimentation was about to get a lot more gnarly.

PART TWO

Tiny Experiments: Year Two

– healing –

The Self-Trust Experiment

As a doula, I have an exquisite trust in women's bodies to birth. I believe that the great majority of births do not actually require the assistance of medical intervention, and I have a deep sorrow for the fact that we have created and live in a culture that believes that birth is dangerous, that women's bodies are faulty and require assistance to birth, and that undermines women's trust in their ability to do what obviously — *because we are all here on this planet right now* — they are born being able to do. Made for it. Perfect.

The distrust in women's bodies that I see in the context of birth is mirrored in the Diet Culture, and, truly, in regards to women's bodies, full stop. *Not to be trusted.*

When we cannot trust our bodies, we look externally for our understanding of how they work. We look to diet books, personal trainers, yoga instructors, doctors, nutritionists, naturopaths, massage therapists, and everyone *but ourselves.* We seek rules and guidelines to follow.

In birth, the risk of trusting the body and being wrong is mortal. Self-trust and intuition and careful attunement are nebulous, and coupled with our fear of the worst outcome imaginable, we turn to what feels more certain: rules, guidelines and policies.

So it is, in many ways, with our relationship to fat. When our self-trust is shaky, and when faced with the shame of fatness in our culture, and with the belief we've come to hold about fatness being unhealthy, our fear of trusting that our bodies will tell us what to eat and what not to eat, when we're hungry and when we're full, is no less mortal than the fears many have come to associate with birth.

The concept of self-trust is conflated with the relationship that most of us, myself included, have with our bodies. We live in a world that really only requires us to function from the neck up. We take in a myriad of stimulation from the eyes, ears, nose and mouth from the minute we wake until our very last moment of consciousness at the end of the day. We process that information in our brain, and most of the output that is required of many of us who live a fairly sedentary lifestyle after that processing is the movement of our mouths and the rapid dance of our fingertips.

It's hard to have trust in something you don't even have a *relationship* with.

Rather than *tuning in* to our bodies to hear the messages they are sending us, we continue to live *tuned out*, and blame our bodies for not giving us a sign that they are unhealthy or unhappy. And as such, our distrust lives on.

I started to wonder: what would happen if I could trust myself? If I were "allowed" to eat whatever I wanted and move whenever I felt the urge, would I just turn into an impulsive Nutella-scarfing maniac? This was my fear. How would I trust myself to choose foods that were good for my body? Is self-trust too much to ask in a culture within which manufactured convenience foods are marketed just as fervently as diets? What about the idea that sugar is addictive? How can I just *trust myself* when my go-to indulgence is considered by many to be *an actual addiction?*

Self-trust expert Sheryl Paul says, "the minute we decide that there is a 'right' thing that we 'should' do — trust becomes impossible; *from that belief, there is nothing but fear."* She continues, "In practice, self-trust is *only* possible when we *reject* the notion of 'right choice' or 'right outcome,' and instead, focus on being in *authentic relationship* with ourselves — focus on the present-moment focus of self-connection — without the blinding pressure of needing the resulting outcome to look a certain way. Self-trust flows freely when we practice *letting go of outcomes* with food and body, and instead, commit our attention to our intuitive, present-moment needs; the ongoing process of exploring and being curious about ourselves and our desires; getting to know ourselves — checking in with ourselves; and being in *ongoing relationship* with that very thing we so badly want to trust — our bodies and our intuition — with *no goal in mind* other than the joy of relationship and connection itself."

What would happen if I could trust myself?

This question continued to play on my mind, and although it brought tumbling with it the very real fears of gaining weight and losing control, I felt deeply compelled to test it.

One of the first steps in the process of intuitive eating is to rid oneself of the diet mentality. Along with this is permission to *go wild.* To eat everything you'd never allowed yourself before, to get rid of the rules. For many, including myself, this phase starts out a little bit terrifying, and then becomes *really really awesome.*

I started out with a very, very large jar of Nutella.

I ate the whole thing. With a spoon. In the span of about two days.

Not feeling guilty about it felt amazing. I gave myself full permission to eat it, and I actually enjoyed it.

I noticed that I didn't eat it all at once. I would have a few spoonfuls at a time, and then without really thinking about it at all, without a dialogue of "too much" and "out of control," I would seemingly quite unconsciously just put the lid back on the jar and put it away.

Once that jar was finished, I bought another one.

I ate that too.

And then the next week, when I passed the jars of Nutella in the grocery store, I kept on walking.

They said this would happen. The intuitive eating gurus that I had been soaking up wisdom from, that is. They said that eventually, when I let go of the dieting mentality, I would have an experience of *habituation* when it came to the foods that I had restricted and then had subsequently triggered overeating for me in the past. In short, if I allowed myself to eat what I wanted, the allure of the forbidden would begin to wear off, and what was once manna from heaven would become…just food.

Along with this revelation in spreadable chocolate, I noticed that I actually had very clear preferences about my food. I think I had always known this somehow, but as a larger-bodied person I realized that I also had a schema of myself who *could not be controlled* around food.

I realize now that this was probably true, in a way, but not because I'm a lesser person than those who have more self-restraint, or because I'm flawed in some way, but rather because I had lived in a perpetual state of restricted eating that caused me to look at anything I considered taboo (aka delicious) like a bloodthirsty wolf.

But here I was, quite deliberate, in fact, about my food choices. Red meat: not my favourite. In summer, savoury breakfasts with cucumber and red onion and Swiss cheese. In winter, soft scrambled eggs. Only the best chocolate. My husband has always teased me about my reluctance to eat anything before I know *exactly* what I want to have. I'll wilt with hunger before I eat something I don't really want. I noticed that when I went to eat at a restaurant, sometimes I wanted a side of onion rings, but just as often, I wanted salad. I noticed that I didn't always want dessert. (whaaaaat???). I noticed every. single. time I chose not to finish something — a bag of chips, a slice of cheesecake — not because I was being regimented or controlling in some way, but because it just didn't taste good enough to continue, or because I was satisfied with what I had already eaten. I realized that I actually felt much more satisfied after a simple home-cooked meal of pan-fried fish, rice and vegetables than after most take-out meals. I found that since having my son, I had an allergic reaction to alcohol and a very unpleasant reaction to caffeine, both of which were adverse enough to almost completely remove my desire to consume these things.

These preferences were a glimpse into self-trust for me, especially when I decided to label them *intuitions*. Perhaps, in fact, these preferences weren't merely quirks of mine, but *messages from my body*.

The Intuitive Eating Experiment

In so many ways, I've spent the vast majority of my life divorcing myself from my body. Whether it was by adhering to externally-constructed rules about my food intake and exercise or just trying to survive being fat in a thin world by drawing attention to all the amazing things I could do with my *mind*, I have been in a state of mind-body-emotion disconnection for a long time.

The extent to which I had, at least since my last formal diet several years ago, lost awareness of my food choices and their impact on my body became apparent in my food tracking experiment. I didn't realize, until it was on paper, how often I ate out, for example, or that caffeine made me feel like crap. I realized that I still had a long way to go before I was truly listening to my body and its needs when it came to my food choices.

I decided to re-visit the concept of intuitive eating. When I had read the *Intuitive Eating* book earlier in my journey, I just wasn't ready for it. It sounded okay, but when I read it I also perceived there to be a lot of rules within the subtext of the book that made me wonder whether it was just another diet. I came to realize that wasn't necessarily the case, and that I had been — ha! — intuitively pursuing intuitive eating in many ways since.

I began regularly seeing my naturopath friend, Dr. Jen, who had become an intuitive eating expert, and I read the *Intu-*

itive Eating Workbook, a recently-published cohort to the *Intuitive Eating* book that helped me to see the process I wanted to follow, step-by-step.

At my first consultation with Dr. Jen, I shared with her the myriad ways in which I was *so done* with ever dieting again, which she assured me was the first step in the intuitive eating process. She gave me a couple of questionnaires to complete, and they affirmed it: I had stopped placing moral value on my food choices, stopped feeling guilty about and punishing myself for those choices. I had done some desensitization experiments (remember all that Nutella?) and truly felt like there were very few foods I wasn't "safe" around (you know that feeling… that bag of chips isn't safe in the cupboard with me in the house). It turned out that my initial experiments in self-trust were actually some of the first steps in the process of the intuitive eating approach. Essentially, intuitive eating started out, for me, as just letting myself eat whatever I wanted to eat, and in whatever quantity I wanted to eat it.

This process felt like I was *rinsing out* years and YEARS of restricted eating. The intuitive eating book poses that we each have "a trigger food" — a food that we regularly binge on, or crave, or punish ourselves for eating. I felt that, for me, *every* food was a trigger food. My love of food is *based on* variety, experimentation, and novelty, and so one minute the trigger food might be Nutella, and the next, Maltesers. The next time I would go to the grocery store, I'd be hunting for a bag of chips, or a block of cheese to melt over everything in sight. My foodie self was *dedicated* to seeking out variety and excitement in my foods, and forbiddenness was *very exciting* to me.

Dr. Jen assured me that this was normal, and that everyone goes through the experience of breaking up with dieting differently, and for different amounts of time. She described the process as being like a pendulum that has been held up in the trappings of restriction for so long, it needs to swing completely the other way — into the somewhat dangerous-feeling realm of *going crazy with food* — before settling back into the middle, where attuned, intuitive eating happens, and food is more neutral than it ever used to be. This is also the point at which research has found people find what's called the metabolic "set point." The set point is the weight at which a person falls most naturally. It has a window of fluctuation by a fairly consistent — but different for everyone — amount of weight, but generally, with the support of intuitive and unrestricted eating, remains the same.

Soon enough, and just like the *Intuitive Eating* principles promised, I stopped feeling so crazy around food. I could *very honestly*, without a single ounce of restrictive thinking, pass by the Maltesers in the candy aisle. I could buy a bag of chips, eat a few, and put them away when they tasted too salty or started stinging my lips, knowing that I could always come back to the bag for more, later that day, or even later that week.

This didn't always happen, of course, and I don't expect it ever will, completely. Sometimes, as the principles of *normal eating* posit, the food in front of me was *so* delicious, or *wouldn't* be available to me again, and it made me want to eat the whole thing, even if I was feeling really full. And I did, and I either noticed that feeling that full didn't feel worth having eaten the food, or I felt really freakin' satisfied. *Either way, it was okay.*

This is where, for me, the intuitive eating principle of *"discovering the satisfaction factor"* came in. I noticed that I had a propensity to eat all of the food that was put in front of me, whether it was satisfying or tasted good or not. I had a habit of seeking out sweet foods after meals and eating them, whether they were satisfying or not. But gradually, I found I regularly forgot about the treats laying around the house that I had purchased, and had had the miraculous experience more than once of leaving things like cheesecake half-eaten on my plate because I was full, or because it didn't taste as good as I thought it would. My natural preferences were to cook and eat fairly "healthy" meals. Sometimes I would let myself get too hungry or too full, but I started to be able to observe these occurrences non-judgmentally, and as my sense of scarcity around food dissipated, so did the occasions upon which I was unable to honour my hunger and fullness.

As I continued to explore intuitive eating with my naturopath, I delved into the realm of emotional eating. Though I agreed with Isabel Foxen Duke and the philosophy of normal eating that emotional eating didn't need to be demonized, I did notice that there were certain times that I was less intuitive and more emotional about my eating. One of those times was when I was craving connection with another person. I regularly used food as a way to connect with others, partially because it feels nurturing, and partially, if I'm being honest, because sharing in an indulgence with someone made me feel less shame than if I were indulging by myself. I found I also would "treat myself" to foods when I was having a bad or busy day. As I worked with Dr. Jen, I started to realize, though, that I was having those days more often than not. At this time, I was not getting enough sleep, trying to cram too many things into my schedule, and generally feeling somewhat drained by parenting. I often sought a pick-me-up — usually in the form of a fancy coffee or some chocolate — to make me feel better. In a way, I was seeking food as a comfort, and very often doing so as a proxy for pleasure when my life was not feeling pleasurable. I also noted a lot of shame still remaining when I ate, especially in front of or with other people. I would avoid going for seconds of a meal, even if I was still hungry, worried about what people might think. I would "pose" as a "healthy eater" when eating in social situations, particularly among people I didn't know well — not taking a dessert or taking a smaller portion, lest people think I was *fat because I overate….obviously*. Finally, I also noticed that I would use food to enhance my pleasure of celebration-worthy occasions. It was as though I couldn't just enjoy, say, getting an article published in a magazine, but that I had to connect the occasion with food as a way to reward and celebrate my accomplishment as well.

Discovering these very specific emotional triggers for non-intuitive eating was helpful, and I began to develop a non-judgmental awareness of the occasions on and reasons for which I ate in an un-attuned way. I still very often chose chocolate over *feeling my feelings*, but I learned to identify *how* I'm feeling, and in doing that, I began to be able to create a moment — *even just a small pause* — where I could make a choice about what I wanted to do with that feeling.

In addition, I learned that perhaps moreso than emotional eating, I'm vulnerable to what Resch and Tribole call "attunement disruptors." Attunement disruptors are anything that inhibit the ability to listen to one's body. Busyness and a lack of self-care are attunement disruptors. So is eating with a kid on your lap, or making said incredibly picky kid a meal of scrambled eggs in the middle of eating your own dinner. No? Just me? Resch and Tribole say that, in this case, "you may feel full but if you didn't experience the pleasures of your meal, you may still have a profound desire to continue eating to experience those joys."

Yup.

Also, eating while distracted lessens the habituation effect of repeated exposure to food, and makes a person less able to tune into how their body is feeling. Meaning, if I'm distracted while I eat a piece of milk chocolate, I'm less likely to notice if it's starting to taste too sweet, or if my tenth bite is still as or less satisfying than my first.

I had a few other revelations as I explored intuitive eating. I realized that few foods *don't* feel good in my body. I had an inkling of this after my tracking experiment, where I noticed that I had great energy, was regular, and generally felt healthy. Overeating did *not* feel good for me, but I didn't or didn't always want to stop myself from doing so. Within the paradigm of normal eating, this is all okay, but the intuitive eating gurus would ask me to invite the question "would I choose to feel that way again?" Sometimes I would; sometimes not. It depended.

The final principle of intuitive eating is one of gentle nutrition. In essence, it means that despite the fact that we can eat whatever we want and shouldn't have rules about food and restriction, vegetables are still good for us. We can shape our meals to be more satisfying and satiating, say, by using basic nutrition guidelines and including fats and proteins with carbo-hydrates. Gentle nutrition is the edict I adopt when I create meal plans: I create plans that are exciting and non-restrictive, but that are generally healthy and include foods that my body likes and needs in order to feel good.

My entire exploration of intuitive eating made me real-ize that, more than anything, my work was not so much intu-itive eating itself, but rather the work of nourishing the condi-tions for intuitive eating to occur: that is, to engage in the most basic self-care, planning and attunement to my body's needs so that I could *allow my intuition to do what it was already doing, but in a way that I could tap into more readily.* Ironically, as my understand-ing of body respect and acceptance matured, I was coming back around to where I started on this whole journey: with honouring my body's most basic requirements for water, hy-giene, sleep, and joyful movement.

The Adventure Experiment

Adventure has long been the way that I prove my ability to myself. My relationship with adventure is a complicated one, with roots in my history of overexercise, and in a thread of "not enough" that is woven through the fabric of my self-doubt. And so for a good long time, after I discovered, on that whitewater rafting trip many years ago, that *my body could do cool things,* and that doing cool things with my body made me feel good, my desire for adventure was also about proving my ability not just to myself, but to the world, as well. It was deeply conflated with my belief that the world saw my fat body as *incapable,* and I wanted to prove them wrong.

Nevertheless, my desire to pursue adventure does continue to have a hold on me, but I've gained the wisdom to know when that desire comes from my darker compulsions, from my need for recognition and validation from external sources. I have gained the wisdom, after years of overexercising, to know when something isn't right for my body; I've lost the desire — *or ability* — to push myself into doing things that don't feel good, or are potentially harmful. The "light" side of my love of adventure is my sense of accomplishment when I set myself to a challenging or novel task, and then achieve it.

Having children sent my sense of adventure into a tailspin. I had become accustomed to extreme endurance events and traveling to foreign countries to satisfy my urge for adventure, and having babies often meant that the biggest adventure I engaged in was leaving the house without a diaper bag. Especially with my first child, leaving her for longer than about three hours while exclusively breastfeeding wasn't really an option. Also, as I learned when I registered to do the swim portion of an Ironman four months postpartum, not only my schedule but my new postpartum body, loose ligaments and weakened ab muscles and all, had a different idea about what I was now capable of as an adventurer.

But, when my youngest child was nearly three, I decided it was finally time to adventure once more.

I was nervous as I slowly plodded down the pebble beach with a fifty pound backpack on my back. The weight on my back and the muscle compensation I had to do to walk across such unsteady ground caused me to get more winded than I had expected. All kinds of negative self-talk flooded my mind as I wondered how I would possibly do a three-day, fifty kilometre hike across terrain that was about to become much, much more challenging than this.

I had wanted to do this trip for years. Too busy having and nursing babies, I had had to put it off, year after year. This time, the point at which I had been on my journey toward body acceptance for almost a year and a half, felt like the perfect opportunity. Could I show myself that my weight didn't actually matter when not measured up against societal norms but against my *ability* instead? Could I Hike While Fat? Could I fully engage in and enjoy the opportunity to test my body, witness amazing natural wonders, and experience the deep back woods, in the body that I inhabit?

It turns out, I could. A thousand times over, I could. Though those first steps on the pebble beach were challenging, and hiking with a pack that heavy was new to me, I soon hit a stride, and all the motivational thinking and goal-setting that had gotten me through endurance events in the past kicked in like it had never left me.

The first day of hiking made me realize that the trail wasn't going to spit me out the other side of it without a fight, though. What I had thought would be an "easy" twelve kilometre first day of hiking took over nine hours. The elevation gains and losses slowed me to a pace that, when I hiked Kilimanjaro, was referred to in Swahili as "pole pole," or very, *very* slow. I leaned hard on my hiking poles, plunging them into the earth to help leverage myself and my pack up steep inclines, and all the while, what started out as a heavy mist became a thundering rain that wouldn't release me from its torrent for the entire three day excursion.

Nevertheless, and to my surprise, I found myself getting stronger and stronger as the days went on. The rising water levels caused what would normally be trickles of water running across the trail to turn into raging waterfalls, some of which, when I crossed them, rose up to my thigh and threatened to loosen my footing and sweep me out toward the ocean. But I didn't waver: I waded through, and kept going, watching the water bubble *out* of my Gore Tex hiking boots with each step. On the final day and during the last few kilometres, my gear was twice as heavy as it was on the first day, now completely waterlogged from three days of rain. Despite this, I actually picked up my pace significantly, finishing the last leg of the journey with ease.

I almost don't have words for how healing this was for my relationship with my body. So many of the things that I think of as being "me" fell by the wayside when I had children, and so did my belief that my body was capable of doing the things that made me feel like "me." This journey brought me full circle once more, as though I needed a more dramatic, stark demonstration of my body's *ability* than I was able to achieve in my usual, everyday life.

The pursuit of adventure and the affirmation of my ability is something that I now hold as a priority in my life. A few weeks after this hike, I went zip lining, navigating a challenging outdoor obstacle course suspended fifty feet in the air. I got certified in Wilderness Remote First Aid, became a certified Hike Leader, and started leading even more challenging wilderness quests with my clients. My intention became to incorporate ways of reminding myself of and testing my ability on a regular basis, to honour my love of adventure, which allows me to feel joy in what my body can do.

The Yoga Teacher Training Experiment

"Body acceptance starts where you are and begins to move first not toward love but toward neutral. Because when you're in neutral, you're IN your body. You're EMBODIED, moving through the world, doing your thing…It's less feeling something about my body and more feeling something IN my body."

— Anna Guest-Jelley, *Curvy Yoga*

I had wanted to do my yoga teacher training for *years* before I finally decided it was time. I have had a yoga practice since the ripe old age of about fifteen, when I did yoga in the elementary school gym with a bunch of my mom's friends and the hippie lady who was the only yoga instructor in town. Yoga wasn't very cool back then, and my primary preoccupation in class as the youngest participant by several decades was trying not to laugh when the ladies would pass gas in child's pose.

I spent the next twenty years in an on-again, off-again relationship with yoga. I practiced regularly in my first year of university, where I found a class taught by yet another hippie lady in a church basement. I attended with my best friend and was reminded the comforts of home as I twisted myself deeply into postures that the rest of the class, consisting primarily of elderly women and the church minister, game for anything, couldn't do. It would have been easy for me, as a young university student, to dismiss the practice as being not cool enough for me, but I found it deeply comforting as I navigated homesickness and the identity shift from child to woman with the matronly instructor guiding me.

I found another class in my second year of university, and my best friend and I trundled to that one – a dynamic, sweaty Astanga practice that pushed both of us to our limits. As I began to establish myself as *someone who exercised,* this class suited my reluctance to spend time moving my body in any way that wouldn't result in a satisfying calorie burn.

In the years I challenged my body in doing triathlons and competitive sports, I would do yoga in my living room once a week as a way to thank my body for its effort. I did the poses my body wanted to do, intuitively, and this was my first foray into yoga-as-nourishment.

It didn't last long, and I became a devotee of hot yoga and all things sweat, effort, and fancy postures.

My feelings about my body in yoga were fairly neutral in the beginning of my practice, but began to change as yoga became more mainstream and as my own body started to change. During my late twenties, practicing regularly in the hot studio, I was able to "keep up" with the thin, lithe women on the mats around me, but something about that began to shift. As yoga became more corporatized and my Instagram feed gradually filled with skinny blondes contorting themselves into complex poses, I busied myself with having children and trying to Lose the Baby Weight. My experience of yoga class became increasingly dissonant: I began to feel like yoga might not be *for me* anymore. I was almost always the fattest woman in the class, and I began to feel deep shame, just for my presence there.

I would often leave my yoga classes feeling more loathing and hatred toward my body than when I walked in. Yoga class became the place where I had to go toe to toe with the amount of weight I had gained in recent years: there was nowhere to hide it in my Lululemon gear, and there were a great many poses — forward folds and inversions, especially — where I would feel as though I were being choked by own fat. I would try to maintain what I *believed* was the integrity of the pose despite the fact that it was limiting the circulation of oxygen to my body and actually causing a fight or flight response — basically the opposite of what's supposed to happen in yoga.

I can't entirely say what made me think that *this* was the right time to sign up for my yoga teacher training. Going to yoga classes had begun to feel so terrible to me (and, let's face it, I was so busy mom-ing) that I no longer had a regular practice. I had always wanted to do a YTT, but I assumed that I would have to learn how to do tricky poses like headstands and handstands first. I also had wanted, in the past, to do yoga teacher training so that I would have another facet of my business to offer. But now, I knew I wanted something different.

I wanted to rediscover my body.

I wanted to use my body as a way of relating in the world, rather than always relying on the power of my mind.

I felt like I was limiting myself, in some way, by shutting down experiences that involved my body and its ability: I was preventing myself from experiencing the fullness of life available to me because I was making assumptions about whether or not my body could partake in these experi-

ences, but also about what others would think if I attempted to partake in these experiences. Yoga teacher training was just one of these things.

A few different experiences began to shift my beliefs around my ability to undertake a teacher training, and to be a yoga instructor. I met a few yoga teachers who I secretly believed probably couldn't do a handstand either, and so I felt emboldened by their presence. I found other fat yoga instructors on social media, like Dana Falsetti and Jessamyn Stanley, and they made me feel like if they could do it, so could I. Mostly, I found the right instructor — one who helped me realize that I could receive all the benefits of yoga in poses that were entirely accessible to me no matter what shape my body had, and who taught me that yoga is actually *not* supposed to be predominantly a physical practice.

I remember the day I finally worked up the courage to email her and ask her about the training. I nervously explained to her that I didn't know how to do any fancy poses, and that my practice had actually been waning in recent years. I distinctly remember feeling as though I wanted to give her an easy way to tell me No. Not this year. Not in this body. Not with me.

But she didn't. She wrote back something about my prana — the life force energy that exists in all of us, which shifts and flows as a result of yoga — and welcomed me with open arms.

The revelation that yoga isn't meant to be as much of a physical practice as I had come to believe still reverberates for me. Although I had had a yoga practice for over twenty years and realized intellectually that yoga was, indeed a spiritual, devotional practice, I had, like so many of us, become completely swept up in the current perception of yoga that lives, most demonstrably, on Instagram, in the form of skinny blonde women standing on their heads on beaches. This perception was subtly but powerfully reinforced in the yoga classes I had been attending at my local studio, and I had begun to believe it.

Interestingly, in fact, Anna Guest-Jelley, the founder of the *Curvy Yoga* movement and author of the book of the same name, talks often about the fact that most modern-day yoga teachers are not even *trained* to understand how it feels to do yoga in a larger body (or in any differently abled body, for that matter), and though they often know how to modify poses to accommodate injury, they are not aware of what might be done to adjust poses so that they are most comfortable and impactful for larger bodies. The cycle perpetuates: when fat people are not represented or feel uncomfortable in yoga classes, they are less likely to advance into teacher trainings. As such, yoga is a practice that has become something that is taught by and *for* smaller-bodied individuals. That's one of the reasons Guest-Jelley's company does *Curvy Yoga* teacher trainings. When I read the *Curvy Yoga* book, which is partially a history of Guest-Jelley's own journey toward yoga and body acceptance and partially a yoga "how to" book, my mind was blown. I had never thought of *moving my belly fat out of the way* when I wanted to do a forward fold. I had *never thought* of widening my legs in child's pose to accommodate my size. I didn't realize I could use a strap to hold my breasts in shoulder stand so that I didn't feel like I was going to smother myself. It was like a giant permission slip to stop obsessing about how my body looked and assuming it didn't belong in a yoga studio, and *just get on with it.*

As my training progressed, I became even more aware of the purpose of yoga as a way to use the physical body as a way to influence one's mental, emotional and energetic experience. I learned that even the simplest poses could achieve that effect; I learned that my physical asana practice was not an end in and of itself but merely a tool for deeper self-connection.

My yoga teacher training instructor was just as matter-of-fact about my body and what it could do as the osteopath that I had begun to see — the one who just dug around in my belly looking for my organs, with no judgement toward the fat they were buried in. It gave me the freedom to be just as non-judgemental and matter-of-fact about my body, myself. I didn't feel the same longing as I once had when I gazed over at my fellow students and saw that their bodies could do different things than mine. I was solely focused on the experience of my *own* body, and I began to see that, in many ways, though the external orientation of the poses I was doing sometimes looked different, my internal experience was often very much the same as my counterparts.

I witnessed this most starkly when I embarked on the forty-day daily yoga and meditation practice that was a part of my training. During this time, I *felt* the way my body was both a mirror for and a gateway to my mind, my emotions and my spirituality. I saw how my struggles to slow down in my busy day-to-day life showed up on my mat, and I would notice myself hurrying to finish my daily poses without checking in with how they felt in my body. I witnessed what happened when I allowed myself to soften and pause. I was healed by the freedom I felt to modify my practice on any given day and *in any given moment* to reflect what my body could do, and what it needed most. I *felt* the way that movement with breath could impact me at an energetic and physiological level, and every so often, in meditation at the end of a powerful practice, I was able to experience the potential my body has as a tool for allowing me to access the divine – that inexplicable and nebulous feeling of "oneness" that those who have tasted it spend a lifetime yearning for.

This is where my heart breaks a little. My heart breaks for all the times I denied myself the opportunity to access a deeper self-knowledge and a glimpse of the infinite because I had been in denial of my body. I had been living ashamed of the very instrument I was gifted with so that I could know wonder, and mystery, and awe, and something greater than myself.

I've settled into a new way of thinking about yoga. I've lost interest in the studio yoga practice that I believed qualified and validated me as a yogi. I see my mat as a place to touch into what's happening below my shoulders, and I have the tools to use yoga to shift the energy that I bring to my life, and to the world around me. I have revitalized my meditation practice, and it's another opportunity I take to check in with myself, to internalize my focus. Although I'm not sure what *teaching* will look like for me from here on out, I like the idea of offering people the opportunity to see and experience yoga in the way that I've been able to. I like the idea of perhaps contributing to a shift in the conversation about what yoga is, and *who it's for.*

My Purpose for my Body

I have long loved the work and writings of Danielle LaPorte. One particular concept that she explored in one of her blog posts resonated with me deeply. She asked the question: what is your purpose for money? At the time, I was in the middle of considering a massive career change that included giving up a healthy, salaried income with benefits in exchange for a lesser-paid position at a non-profit. I noticed myself becoming quite embroiled in the number that would be my new salary, and noticed that I had had a value about money and income that hadn't fully surfaced until I had considered this career change.

The question "what is your purpose for money?" is not about how *much* money you want to make, but rather the deep and abiding purpose you have for making that money. It's about naming the handful of things that you want to *do* with your money. Asking this question of myself allowed me to see through all of my made-up stories about how much money I needed or wanted to make per year, and caused me to really ask if my money was achieving what I wanted it to achieve for me. Realizing my purpose for money made me realize that that purpose could actually be fulfilled on a much lower salary, and with a reprioritization of some of my expenditures that didn't align with that purpose.

The power of asking this question made me want to ask the same question about my body. I was taken aback to realize that I hadn't truly engaged with this way of thinking about my body before. Asking *"what is my purpose for my body"* was a massive wake-up call. I had spent the last twenty or more years obsessed with the appearance and subsequent social acceptability of my body, without actually tuning into what I wanted to achieve with my body, in my body. How my body could *serve* me, and serve the purpose I had for my life.

Because surely fitting back into my pre-motherhood pants or enjoying the reflection I saw in shop windows as I walked down the street couldn't be the reason I was put here on this earth in this particular physical form, no?

When I asked myself "what is your purpose for your body," along with "what do you really want here?," and "how do you want to feel?," the answer came swiftly and confidently.

I want to be able to experience life's joys.

In the past, perhaps my response to this question would have been to "be healthy," but truthfully, I don't know what healthy actually *feels* like. What does *healthy* allow me to do? My sense was that healthy was actually a thinly-veiled manifestation of my acculturated beliefs that healthy meant thin. I *am* healthy. And I'm fat.

So what do I really *want?* What do I want my body to achieve for me?

I want to be able to jump into the lake and swim to the other side. I want to feel the cold water around my body and see the sun sparkling off the waves as I turn my head to breathe. I want my body to be able to feel the joyous embraces

165

and soft little kisses of my two beautiful children, whom, incidentally, my body created, birthed and nourished, all by itself. I want my body to allow me to travel all over the world and experience the tastes, smells, sights and sounds of new cultures. I want to fly down hills on my bicycle, experience deep peace in meditation, and feel the excited terror of a wave barrelling toward me as I prepare to jump to my feet on my surfboard. I want my body to allow me to know the exquisiteness of a perfectly-set creme brûlée, to delight in the pleasure of cracking a perfectly caramelized crust of sugar with my spoon. I want to feel my toes curling into dewy grass, and my hands to know when the tomatoes are ripe for picking. I want to use my hands to hold the hands of those I love, and to press firmly on the backs and legs of the labouring women I support; I want my hands to offer comfort. I want to feel wind in my hair, and smell lilacs in the spring. I want my body to know the pleasure of a flowing, floral dress tickling my legs as I walk. I want to know what it is to be held and to feel deeply supported and cared for. I want to hear the peeper frogs on a cool spring night, and my daughter saying "I love you times infinity times a hundred million galaxy universes!" I want my body to help me learn its wisdom, to guide my intuition with the feeling in my gut and to walk me through the forest as I seek clarity.

This is what it is to be able to experience life's joys.

This is my purpose for my body.

And every. single. one. of these things are possible no matter the shape of my body. Every single one.

I have to wonder, what else is there? We are each given a body with which to experience this earthly realm. Truly, we have no idea why we've been granted the physical form we've been granted. We are each so entirely different in so many ways, and we were, for the most part, made that way. And so what more do we have to do, truly, than accept that form and allow it — *truly allow it* — to give us the *gift* of the human experience we were meant to, and deserve to, enjoy?

The Healing: Hosting the Reunion

My tiny experiments in what it might be to accept, respect, and possibly even love my body brought me to a very different place than I expected.

I have lived my entire life believing (and I still live in a culture that believes) that the only way I would be able to accept my body would be, ironically, to change it.

I never, ever imagined that I might be able to accept my body in a form that has been so wholeheartedly deemed *unacceptable* by women's magazines, the patriarchy, health professionals, the fashion industry, and just about every single person I interface with on a day-to-day basis.

I am so grateful that my tiny experiments veered me into the only direction, I now realize, that could ever bring me body acceptance: the full and deep knowledge that there is nothing I can *or want to* do to change my body.

But the road I took to get here left me scarred. The lashings of self-hatred I've dealt myself have left well-worn neural pathways that still activate every time I stand in front of the mirror. The marks left by the hurtful words of others, both hurled and insinuated, rival the marks left by my widening thighs and softening belly.

All of this has left me sitting in the complexity of both pain and hope, loathing and love, surrender and fear.

I feel tentatively able to conceive a future where I see and treat my body as a sacred vessel.

I also feel a deep desire to heal the pain of what it has been to live in this body, to navigate living in this body in the world, for the last thirty-six years.

Part of this healing has happened already, as I've engaged in the process and writing of this book.

And part of it will happen as I continue to, as Glennon Doyle says, *host the reunion* between my body and my mind and soul.

I had to come to a place where I could believe that my body was worth living in, was worth paying attention to and had something valuable to say, before I could begin the process of reuniting the lost parts of myself.

And now, I'm here.

PART THREE:

Reclamation

My journey thus far has brought me here: to a place where body acceptance, respect and love feels somewhat secondary to the possibility of Reclamation. Of reuniting myself with my body, of reclaiming my relationship with my physical form in a way that the conditioning of my past and the culture I'm surrounded in would have me deny at all costs.

And so, still, I forge on.

Reunited: 41 Things I Know About My Body

1. My toes are prehensile: I can pick up toys off the floor with them like a goddamn monkey.
2. I like the way my toes look. I usually keep my toenails natural and I like the way they fit perfectly into my Birkenstocks in the summer.
3. My feet are wide, like paddles. They're hard to find shoes for, but I like to think that they make me a better swimmer.
4. My feet have walked me all over the world: they have been barefoot at the Taj Mahal, sitting, dressed in flowing scarves and talking to a local family about our respective lives. They have been fitted into scuba fins and have propelled me into caves with sharks, toward dinner-table sized turtles, swimming over shipwrecks hundreds of years old. My feet have run the pavement in a small town in Vietnam and biked to a war monument in Cambodia. These feet have curled up on the floor with Romanian orphans. They have paced the halls of a hospital while I laboured with my first baby, and while I supported other women to birth theirs. They have

run marathons, and half marathons, and played football and swum and biked more kilometres than I can count.

5. My ankles have been sprained many times. When I sprain them, I get a dark purple bruise that streaks through the hollow between my ankle bone and the sole of my foot.

6. Despite their many injuries, my ankles are one of my favourite places on my body — not necessarily for their strength or what they do for my body, but because, simply enough, they are conventionally attractive. Easy to love. When my hips widen or my belly feels fuller, my ankles are always the same.

7. I have an om tattoo on my left inner ankle. Now, in my thirties, I have come to realize that its location is actually really culturally offensive. I'm designing a cover-up for it.

8. My calves are lovely. They have always looked strong and toned, even when they've been neglected. They *are* strong, even when they've been neglected. I am confident that they will carry me on big hikes and silently down the stairs as my children sleep. My calves are my favourite feature, to be sure.

9. My knees are a source of nearly constant pain. One of them has been completely dislocated several times playing football, and falling on ice. My knees grind when I climb and descend the stairs, such that I will never be a very good participant in any kind of multi-floor game of hide and seek. It hurts to squat in front of my kids, so that I can look them in the eye when I'm speaking to them. Many times, I can't sit still because it hurts to extend my legs *and* it hurts to bend them. I've found, though, that yoga helps a lot, and so does not doing things that hurt, like running. That took me longer to realize than I'd like to admit.

10. My thighs have always been strong, too. They walk me everywhere, just as reliably as my calves. Since having my kids, the rock-hard lateral muscle I used to run my hand over, just to feel its firmness, has gotten smaller and softened. There is some dimpling along the sides of my thighs that I run my hands over now, too. When I kneel, I notice that my inner thighs gravitate toward the floor in a way they never used to.

11. My butt is wide and flat. It's always been that way, even in various states of tone. I don't mind, so much, that it billows out beside me more now than it used to. My hips feel like something someone might want to hold on to.

12. As I run my hands down the sides of my thighs, they feel different than they once did. Never a place I used to carry weight, the once-smooth skin now has pockets of fleshiness that I am learning to explore. Mostly, I am fascinated.

13. My uterus has conceived, carried and birthed two babies. I feel so blessed that I was able to conceive my children without difficulty, and that my pregnancies were beautiful, powerful experiences. My births were smooth and unmedicated, and left me feeling like I could achieve *anything*. I am so, so deeply grateful for this, for being a woman, for having this potential in my body, for having brought two souls earthside powerfully and perfectly, each in their own way.

14. I bleed on the full moon. Since finally giving up birth control after having my kids, my body has returned to a natural cycle that follows the lunar cycles. This feels like such a deep confirmation of my wildness, my sense of belonging on the earth. Noticing the moon helps me notice my periods; noticing my periods helps me notice the moon. We are inextricably connected. And alongside this awareness, I've grown a deeper awareness of my body's need for rest dur-

ing my bleeding time. I now honour that, slowing down, doing less, taking baths, sleeping more, saving my creativity and my desire to "get things done" for the new moon, when I'm more likely to feel the urge to start projects anew.

15. My body is my children's home. It was their home, quite tangibly, when I carried them in my uterus, where my cells nourished theirs for ten months. But it's *still* their home. My son curls across the softness of my belly when he nurses; my breasts the most comforting thing he knows, even now at the age of three. My daughter tucks herself under my arm and against my belly and legs as I snuggle her to sleep. She is the ultimate snuggler, and it is in my arms where she finds home.

16. The crest of my pelvis — my hips — are a place to rest weary babies and the straps of heavy backpacks. It's a place to put my hands when I'm feeling both confident and self-conscious. There's a place that appears when I lay on my side and gravity pulls the flesh away from my pelvic bone — it's a little bit concave and a little bit vulnerable and a little bit steady and grounded, and it's my husband's favourite place to rest his hand. I like putting my hand there too, as if I were reminding myself of something — my strength, or my femininity, or my sensuality.

17. My belly has always been round: there has never been a time, living in my body, when I can remember firmness or flatness there. During my pregnancies were, ironically, the only times I didn't feel vulnerable showing my belly — the only times I would wear fitted shirts and revel in my profile, when the bodies of my babies stretched my roundness into a more societally-acceptable shape.

18. I have stretch marks that rise up, red and silvery and wide, from my pubic bone up toward my belly button. I didn't see

them forming underneath the growing fundus of my uterus during my second pregnancy; it wasn't until my baby lay sleeping next to me that I knew they were there, and could run my hands over them, feeling they were as foreign to my fingers as the surface of the moon.

19. I feel like my belly must hold a lot of pain, the pain of cruel judgements both spoken and unspoken by myself and others. It is the place that still causes me to shrink back when touched, as if the hands of myself or others on that vulnerable place would somehow make it real, something that I could not hide any longer. Often now, though, I cradle it in my hands. So often, really, that I reach for it almost unconsciously, just to feel that it's there and, perhaps, in my acknowledgement, find some acceptance.

20. Still, though, my belly defines my physical experience of the world in so many ways — it is what defines what clothing I feel good wearing, and, as a result, what clothing, brands, and sizes I can actually buy; in that way, it defines how I present myself to the outside world. I hold a constant awareness of what my belly looks and feels like — of whether my shirt is clinging too tightly to my stomach as I sit down and needs to be pulled away, or how it feels to bend into a yoga pose in which I feel restricted because of my stomach.

21. Someone once said my back was strong, because my vertebrae are tucked deeply between thick, protective muscle, all the way up. I tucked that compliment away in my psyche, and bring it out whenever I need to hear it again.

22. Though I have degenerative disc disorder, I have learned that regular bodywork and yoga help to keep my back from hurting. It used to be that my back would go out every few months, and I would spend several weeks — sometimes

longer — in excruciating pain. I've always been told that I would have to learn to live with this — that there was no cure — and I guess I have.

23. I love the way my lower back feels when I reach my hands there, feeling the paradoxical strength of those muscles, despite my vertebral weakness. I push my palms downward toward the widening of my hips and I feel sturdy, solid.

24. The middle of my back is often so tight that it is sore to the touch. It feels delicious to drape myself over a yoga bolster to allow that part of my body some release. Six years of draping my body over my children as I nursed them, six years of following my passion for writing, hunched over the keyboard of my computer: the tightening of my musculature here, perhaps, a response to the opening that the muscle opposite it — my heart — has done.

25. My mother used to tell me that when I was a baby, she used to marvel at the size of my ribcage and my shoulders — that even then, I had a wide, thick chest and broad shoulders. They joked that I should become a swimmer, and I did. On the rare occasion that I glimpse my bare shoulders in a double mirror, I am in awe of the muscles I see rippling there. Even though my body now holds more flesh under my arms and across my chest than it did when I was a long-distance swimmer, I still hold tremendous strength there. As a younger woman, I used to puff up my chest as I walked, so as to look even broader, even stronger. Maybe I should start doing that again.

26. My breasts have nourished my two children. Perfectly. They've always been more pendulous than perky, but they are perfect nonetheless. And in the last five years, they've been the subject of more adoration than I ever thought

imaginable: my children both love my breasts with unadulterated affection. Rightfully so.

27. My shoulders can carry everything I need to survive for days in the woods. They have carried me, through the water, across oceans, for miles.

28. My shoulders creep up toward my ears when I am feeling stressed out. My eyebrows furrow then, too.

29. They've seen their share of damage, too, my shoulders. I have to be careful about how I sleep, about where I place my hands in the water as I swim, about doing chatturunga in yoga class. Sometimes they hurt.

30. My arms are strong and sinuous. Though they've also gathered more flesh as my body has changed over the years, I marvel in the rippling of muscle as I reach out to grab my baby to stop him from falling, as I held my husband's hand while birthing that baby.

31. I have a tattoo — a simple line — on my wrist: the curve of a cresting wave. It's a reminder of my favourite quote, and the thing I most need to remember, it seems: "save your strength to swim with the tide." It's about surrender, and destiny, and connecting to true power.

32. My fingers know how to type, to play Fur Elise from start to finish on the piano, and to find the chords to my favourite songs on the guitar. They know how to write the words of my heart onto a page or type them into my computer; they are the vehicle for my favourite form of catharsis. My fingers know the feel of my children's soft hair, and the way it feels when my husband interlaces his thick fingers in mine.

33. I touch my chest absentmindedly all the time. I run my fingers across my collarbones when I'm thinking, I press a palm to my heartspace when the words I'm saying come

from there, or when I require a momentary comfort. It grounds me, I think, to feel the steadiness of my shoulders and collarbone swell up into the softness of my breasts.

34. My neck and shoulders have been a source of nearly constant discomfort for me, starting, I believe, in my long distance swimming years, and becoming aggravated the more often I spent time hunched over a nursing baby, or twisted around a small body to offer nourishment in the night. Hot packs and regular massages help.

35. I always used to silently appreciate the fact that my face didn't reflect the size of the rest of my body; I always had a defined jawline and cheekbones. In recent years, I've noticed that I do, in fact, carry more thickness around my jaw, in a way I believed myself immune from. I catch the sight of my face out of the corner of my eye as I pass a mirror, and know that everything changes, even the things I thought would stay the same.

36. My lips know only the most intimate of my relationships. They know what it feels like to touch the soft folds of my toddler's neck, or my daughter's own chapped lips, light and soft, as I kiss her goodbye at school. They know the greatest pleasures — of love and the silkiness of creme brûlée, both.

37. As a teenager, I thought, one day as I sat on a rock near the lake in my hometown, that my eyes were the exact colour of the lake water. Dark, dark blue — blue only upon close inspection. I decided, being a poetic, ruminating teenager, that that was a very. good. thing. I've always thought of the colour of my eyes as being quite special, since then. Like lake water.

38. My eyes don't work very well. I've worn glasses since I was seven years old, and at this point, I'm nearly blind without

them. Sometimes I used to worry that, if my house were to catch fire in the middle of the night, and I were to knock my glasses off my nightstand, I would be helpless to get out of the burning building alive. *That's* how bad my eyes are.

39. I have an eyelid which, as the years of my life have ticked on, has begun to droop. At first it was hardly noticeable, and now I am extremely self-conscious about it. It droops almost to closing when I'm coming home from supporting an all-night birth or have been awake with a sick child; when I'm at my most exhausted. It nearly closes completely when I smile widely, and photos of me always look lop-sided and asymmetrical, at least to me. I have yet to see my droopy eyelid as a quirky physical feature; instead it makes me shy away from the camera, which always seems to capture proof that it exists.

40. My hair has always been one of my best features. Dark blonde with natural highlights, straight and thick with a natural wave. I used to wear it long, down to my waist, all mermaid-like, but it looks just as good cropped or buzzed into a funky short 'do, and it's been red, orange, blue, pink and yellow, too. I have always "led with my hair," in a way — I have used it as a way to express to the world, in a small way, who I am and what I'm about. I've always felt comfortable putting my hair out there, first, for the world to see.

41. My experience of existing physically in the world has — perhaps always — been one of seemingly incompatible dichotomies. Strong and in pain. Soft and muscular. Fat and athletic. Beautiful and not conventionally beautiful. Able and unable. And when I think of my body in that way, I think of it as *just a body*. Just like my osteopath as she works with my physical form *as it is*, in that moment, without

judgment. Just a body, like everyone else has, that works really well in some ways, and not as well in others. That "fits in" with a more socially accepted ideal in some ways, and not in others. That has quirks and faults and strengths that *just are*. There to be dealt with, accepted, celebrated, nourished, honoured, all the same.

"The body is like an earth. It is a land unto itself...The hips, they are wide for a reason, inside them is a satiny ivory cradle for new life. A woman's hips are outriggers for the body above and below; they are portals, they are a lush cushion, the handholds for love, a place for children to hide behind. The legs, they are meant to take us, sometimes to propel us; they are the pulleys that help us lift, they are the anillo, the ring for encircling a lover. They cannot be too this or too that. They are what they are."

— Clarissa Pinkola Estes, *Women Who Run With The Wolves*

The Apology

I am sorry.

I am sorry for all the carrot sticks.

I know you don't like them.

Even when they're dipped in hummus.

I am sorry.

I am sorry for the time I drew, in permanent marker, lines around your middle, around the places I wanted to excise, if only I had a knife.

And for the times I squeezed that flesh so hard my hands hurt and left bruises, wanting some way to release my hatred.

I am sorry for the hatred.

I am sorry for not listening when you were hungry

for food, for touch, for water, for stillness, for movement, for acceptance, for chocolate

I am sorry for not listening when you were full

of tension, of food, of hatred, of longing, of potential

I am sorry for not meeting your needs

or even knowing what they were

or, in fact, acknowledging that you might have them.

You must have felt

like an unmothered child

alone, unloved, trying to survive.

I am sorry for the miles I ran

when you were hurting

I am sorry for running those miles

to punish you

for being the way you were.

I'm sorry for believing someone or something else had the answers

(for believing we *needed answers*)

for assuming you were broken
and for everything that happened when I consulted

everyone but you.

I am sorry for hiding

you

as though you were the representation of everything that was
wrong with me

I am sorry for all the times I tried to transform you into something different

I am sorry for the shame

that I cloaked you in

downcast eyes

tugged clothing

crossed arms

and all.

I am sorry for all those fashion magazines

for cutting out pictures of other women's bodies

and pasting them to my vision boards

I don't buy them anymore.

I am sorry for believing him

when he said you would be perfect if only it weren't for *this part right there*

I'm sorry that I didn't know I should be defending you

rather than being complicit in your degradation.

I am sorry for all the times I tried to squeeze you into jeans that didn't really fit

and for not listening, even when you ached to be released.

And I'm sorry for how I hated you even more

when you didn't fit in

to jeans

or to any of mine or others' expectations about how you should look or how you should be.
(I am sorry for all those shoulds, really)

I am sorry about all the hours I wasted

hating you,

trying to change you,

when I could have been

...I don't know...

changing the world.

I am sorry for trying to keep *both of us* small.

Forgiveness

Every single women's magazine.

Every person who asked when I was due

(when I wasn't pregnant)

The clothing stores that don't carry my size

and all of the places and ways in which I never felt a sense of belonging: the clothing swaps, the yoga classes, every time my lived experience as a fat person went unrecognized and unacknowledged.

I forgive you.

The boyfriend who wished my stomach were smaller

All the men who didn't even consider me worthy of their attention because of the size and shape of my body.

(society, and myself, for the belief that male approval and the "male gaze" is the currency for valuing women's bodies).

I forgive you, too.

Every seemingly offhanded remark during my childhood

"Big-boned."

"She'll grow out of it."

And those of my adulthood

"You're huge."

"You'd be perfect if only…"

"You're plus size, you would know."

I forgive you.

Everyone who has underestimated me

shamed me

been ashamed of me

I forgive you.

I've tried everything to direct your attention to my mind, to my accomplishments, to what I could achieve, physically, *despite being fat,* and I'm no longer willing to do those things

which leaves me here

just fat.

and a whole bunch of other things, too, but also: just as I am. Just what you see, without the distraction of my proving and doing and denying and proving yet again.

I forgive you.

I forgive you.

I forgive you.

What's Still There

"The difference between comfort and nurture is this: if you have a plant that is sick because you keep it in a dark closet, and you say soothing words to it, that is comfort. If you take the plant out of the closet and put it in the sun, give it something to drink, and then talk with it, that is nurture."

—Clarissa Pinkola Estes, *Women Who Run With the Wolves*

The vast majority of this book poured out of me, like a dam of shame and loathing had broken open, like a wound that had been begging for healing for a lifetime.

Until now. The end.

For many months, these final paragraphs remained a mystery to me. I had spent two years coming to a place of deep acceptance and mostly-neutrality when considering the way I felt about my body. But I felt like I couldn't share this journey — couldn't consider it successful, really — until I felt *love* toward my body.

In the time since I began this exploration, though, I came to realize that, when it came to the elusive *body love*, I would remain *seeking*, forevermore. Because belonging in one's own skin is a practice, a daily aspiration, and not an end goal.

But let's face it: I was really hoping this would just end. My struggle, the feelings I feel about living in a large body, would just go away, and I would become one of those brightly-clad curvy, give-no-fucks goddesses that I so admire for their ability to just *show up* in their bodies, just as they are.

I signed up for bellydance class in the hopes of finally becoming that brightly-clad goddess: I thought the class might embolden me with an outward expression of the inward liberation I found in being on this two-year journey. Instead, I found it hard to look at myself in the mirror of the dance studio, and to see how my body looked and moved in comparison to the other, thinner women in the room. I knew to ask for a "plus-size" coin belt with little judgment for the different requirements my body had as compared to the rest of the women in the class, but still, I sized myself up against them, out of habit. I had more neutrality than I have ever had before as I wondered what it must be like to sashay about in a different physical form, but also, I kept my tank top firmly tucked into my leggings, unwilling to witness my belly fat shaking, and especially unwilling to have others witness it too.

During the process of writing this book, I had also imagined that I would have nude photographs taken to complete the process: the ultimate act of a give-no-fucks goddess. And though it took a healthy dose of courage and self-acceptance to even slide my robe off in front of a photographer, I look at those photos with a sometimes baffling combination of awe and fear, joy and sadness.

Sometimes I worry — albeit only sometimes and only very briefly — that actually all of this *acceptance* was a terrible idea and that I will just continue to get fatter and fatter. I wonder if I will ever dance with diets again. Right now I'm confident I won't, but there's also this:

People will continue to ask me if I'm pregnant, as they do and always have done on a freakishly regular basis.

I will still have a hard time finding clothes in stores that cater to smaller bodies.

And I still live in a culture where thin is the ideal, and that ideal is perpetuated over and over, such that nearly every experience I have in the world is somehow marked by it, explicitly or implicitly.

I live in a culture where thin privilege is a *thing*. Where I have a categorically more challenging time navigating through the world because of my size, and where fatness is oppressed. And, in fact, I *don't* want to diminish the work that I did to try to be accepted and fit into the world as a fat person – all those diets and exercise regimes were a part of the emotional (and physical) labour I had to do to feel safe and loved before I had the skills and self-belief to think and do differently. I will never have thin privilege, but even now that I've chosen to stop attempting to have it by changing my body, it doesn't mean that thin privilege doesn't affect me, and that fat discrimination isn't a part of my everyday reality.

And this is hard. Being fat in a thin world is hard to do. And so rather than trying to deny that — and subsequently admonish myself for not being more resilient — I want to acknowledge that fact, honour this challenge in my life, and invite self- compassion for the days when my fatness makes me sad.

This is the complexity I couldn't engage with as I struggled to finish this book with a polished "look at me now" ending.

It's complex, this work of loving my body while living in a culture that tells me I shouldn't. And I can choose the stance I want to take when it comes to living in that culture: I can hide, I can be outspoken, I can turn inward and focus on myself. I can ask myself, when I'm triggered or feeling crappy about my body, what my body wants to be able to feel better about itself. And the answer doesn't always have to be beautiful or militant or empowered. It might sometimes be about self-preservation and doing what works, and I think that's okay.

Anna Guest-Jelley talks about body acceptance and respect as being a practice — like brushing your teeth. She reminds us that we don't struggle with the fact that we need to brush our teeth every day — we just accept it, and we do it. My practice — the one that I've learned from all of this experimentation — is to be *in relationship* with my body, rather than feeling doomed or tethered by it. My intention is to ask myself, as often as I can, what I most *need* — what my *body* most needs — at any given time. And I'm also learning some of my very basic needs, so that I can create a structure of nourishment within my life: hydration, joyful movement, sleep, intuitive eating, meditation, adventure.

To me, this relationship with my body reminds me of the attachment bonds parents create with their children in the early years. Parents' whole purpose, truly, is to meet their children's needs and then gradually teach them to listen to and meet their own. By doing so, especially in the early years, we help our kids create a feeling of safety and security, a sense of knowing that the world is a safe place. From here, they create a schema of "secure base," meaning that their idea of the world as safe, their knowledge that *someone has their back,* allows them to venture out more freely and autonomously into the world. We do this readily for our children, and yet not so much for ourselves. We rarely ask ourselves what we need — *like truly, truly need* — and consequently, we often let others' priorities override our own. In doing this, we subconsciously teach ourselves that we cannot be trusted. We put others before ourselves, and ignore our cues for nurturing, nourishment and attention, disrupting our own attachment bonds *with ourselves.* We erode our internalized sense of self-trust, and then begin, as insecurely attached children do, to withdraw even further, perpetuating the lack of attunement to our basic needs.

So my intention, now, is just to meet my needs. To listen to them, and meet them. And, as a result, to actively engage, on a daily basis, with the work of *hosting the reunion* between my body and the rest of who I know myself to be.

I also know that I do and will continue to do this completely imperfectly. I will not always be "healthy" or feel great. My body will continue to age and change. I will always need to be in relationship to my body and to be reflexive to its *actual* health needs. I will need to be able to look at those needs in a sane way — recognizing that being fat isn't the problem, and my body is no less worthy for being unwell or unable. I want to always remember that there are also seasons to everything, and that sometimes it will be easier to meet my needs, sometimes it will be harder.

This is where I believe the practice of self-compassion enters in. When I am self-compassionate, a tender, loving voice deep within gently reminds me that *I'm okay*. That I'm doing my best, that life sometimes presents challenges, that it's okay to fall short of my own expectations, to fail to meet my needs, and that it's okay to be sad or mad about my body and how I feel in it.

It is with self-compassion that I'm able to release this book into the world, with so many paradoxes and unresolved feelings and with a promise only that there will be more healing yet to be done.

I wanted to be the kind of person who could celebrate the conclusion of this writing process by prancing around naked on a beach somewhere – or even in a locker room somewhere. I sort of wish I *was* that kind of person. I wonder if one day I will be. But this book can't wait for that day. Because I think, in the sharing, my healing is meant to continue, and perhaps yours might too.

Regardless, I think I'm ready, now, to stop writing about my body, and start living in it. I feel I have come to that final phase of the Heroine's Journey, when the time comes to integrate what I've learned and share it with the world.

The Journey Forward: Sacred Body

"may your body be blessed.
may you realize that your body is a faithful and beautiful friend of your
soul.
And may you be peaceful and joyful and recognize that your senses are
sacred thresholds.
May you realize that holiness is mindful, gazing, feeling, hearing and
touching,
May your senses gather you and bring you home,
May your senses always enable you to celebrate the universe and the mys-
tery and possibilities in your presence here."

- John O'Donohue, *Anam Cara*

The realization that is making itself known at the edges of my consciousness, unveiled by my yoga teacher training and the clarity I experienced around my purpose for my body, is that my body is the vessel that is allowing my soul — *that mysterious life force within me that I dance with daily and yet cannot see* — to have an experience on earth. And conversely, my body is actually the *means* through which I can experience the mystery of my spiritual potential because it is, fundamentally, my only vehicle for collecting perceptions, both physical and spiritual. As Anne Bérubé wrote in her book, *Be Feel Think Do,* "often, when we talk about the body in a spiritual context, we don't consider [it] as the primary gateway for the soul's expression. This is experiencing spirituality through the human body."

Put simply, if I'm going to hear the voice of my intuition or some other mysterious guiding force, I'm going to hear it with the ears affixed to either side of my head. If I'm going to see the unbridled joy of what it is to be human, I'm going to see it with my own two eyes as my children run toward me, arms outstretched.

On a personal level, I grieve for the years I spent not understanding this sacred potential in my body, and I now want to choose to embrace the fact that, no matter how it looks or even how I feel about it on any given day, it's the only tool I have through which to know true joy, and experience the divine. It is the tool through which my soul has decided to fulfill its purpose.

And it seems a little foolish to fuck with that.

But this sacred potential goes far beyond the personal, and into the realm of the societal and political – into the ways in which women have been stripped of their power by being stripped of the ability to access their bodies as a power source.

As Sue Monk Kidd says in *The Dance of the Dissident Daughter,*

"Walking into the sacredness of the female body will cause a woman to 'enter into' her body in a new way, be at home in it, honour it, nurture it, listen to it, delight in its sensual music. She will experience her female flesh as beautiful and holy, as a vessel of the sacred. She will live from her gut and feet and hands and instincts and not entirely in her head. Such a woman conveys a formidable presence because power resides IN her

body. The bodies of such women, instead of being groomed to some external standard, are penetrated with soul, quickened from the inside."

On a societal, political level, women taking back autonomy over our physical bodies, which have been systematically violated and devalued, is revolutionary. But taking back our bodies as spiritual vessels is what I believe is required to facilitate not just the dismantling of the oppressive patriarchy, but the *rising of the sacred feminine[3] as well as a culture that honours women, women's knowledge, and women's bodies.* By this I mean: it is one thing to stop our bodies from being controlled and harmed; it is entirely another thing to claim them as sacred.

As Sue Monk Kidd goes on to say about the rising feminine in all of us,

"As a woman...takes back her body...in this act of reclamation she takes back not only her personal physical form but she embodies the sacredness of the feminine for all of us. She begins to make conscious its needs. Through conscious nutrition, exercise, bathing, rest-taking, healing, lovemaking, birthing, and dying she reminds us of the sanctity of the feminine. For many women, including myself, the most sacred moments have been physical ones: being held, making love, nursing a child. Nothing brought me closer to the ecstasy of the sacred than giving birth. The sacred

---

[3] The idea of the sacred feminine is not intended to be gendered, although our culture has come to think of masculine and feminine as the representation of a dichotomy relating to males and females (and thus excluding those who do not identify as such). Rather, the feminine is an archetypal trait that exists in all people. Call it "right brain," call it "yin" – it's an undervalued and yet valuable way of being in the world – one that honours intuition, complexity, compassion, mystery and earth-connection.

dimension is embodied, and the soul of a human being as well as the soul of a culture cannot evolve if the body is not reclaimed and honoured."

And so it is that this work of reclaiming our bodies is both an individual and a collective imperative. This work is – but is also so much more than – about finding jeans that fit and eating whatever you want: this work is about shifting culture and power dynamics and claiming the fullness of your humanity in the face of structures of oppression. It is about dismantling those oppressive structures by opting out of the belief that fatness deems us unacceptable or unworthy in any way.

Though some days the sacred potential of my body escapes me, my deepest wish as I write these final words is that I know my body's *true* purpose, and its potential. May I remember all the ways in which my body has *already* allowed me to access the divine, in the feel of my lips against the folds of my infant son's neck, in the taste of a perfect creme brulée, and in those fleeting moments of stillness when I know my connection to all that is – my infiniteness – because my body was there to perceive it. Exactly as it is.

In this way, even on the days that I may struggle to accept my body, I can say with certainty that *I have reclaimed it.*

ACKNOWLEDGEMENTS

I owe the deepest debt of gratitude to the dozens of women – thought leaders, Instagrammers, podcasters, authors, and activists – who helped me change the way I think about my body and the world my body occupies.

Thank-you to the individuals who supported my personal journey, including but not limited to Dr. Jen Salib-Huber, my naturopath, Heather, my YTT instructor, Monique and Elinor, my bellydance instructors, and DeeDee Morris, whose lens witnessed my unbecoming and becoming once more.

My deepest appreciation to my editor, Renee Hartleib, for helping me to make sure these words said what I wanted them to say, and for giving me the encouragement to put this work out into the world. Also a huge thank-you to Katie: who knew you had such editing skills!

To Katharina Reed, my mentor: words cannot express my gratitude to you as you've called me to my truth and into my power these last seven years. Your eyes on this manuscript shifted the journey significantly for me, even when I thought it was finished, and deepened my thinking and curiosity even further.

To the women I work with and write for: you have been in my mind every step along the way. Though I wrote this book for myself, I wrote it with the cognizance and comfort of knowing that these words might hold meaning for you, too.

Without fully knowing it, you've supported me along this journey.

To Ada and Max: you are what inspires me to keep seeking, to continue healing. You fill my life with joy.

To my husband, Dylan, for the early mornings and the late nights, your patience, your faith in me, and that way you love me no matter what. I know I've taken us on a wild ride: thank you for being my partner through it all.

ABOUT THE AUTHOR

Jessie Harrold is a writer, teacher, coach and doula. Her eclectic mix of skills and interests unite in supporting women + mothers to unearth and reclaim their connection to themselves and their power. Toeing the line between science and magic, the personal and political, Jessie's work explores sovereignty and authenticity, life transition and rites of passage, ecofeminism and earth connection, ancestral skills and restoring the wild feminine.

Jessie holds undergraduate degrees in Neuroscience and Theatre, a Masters of Health Promotion, and life coaching certifications from the Centre for Applied Neuroscience and the Centre for Narrative Coaching and Design. Her qualitative, story-based research on women's experiences navigating health and well-being has won multiple awards and been published in peer-reviewed journals internationally. Her writing has been featured in *Explore Magazine*, Mind Body Green, *Inspired Coach Magazine*, and *International Doula Magazine*.

Jessie offers two online programs – unEARTH and motherSHIFT – and leads pregnancy retreats, and reWILD wilderness quests. She writes prolifically and provocatively on her blog and on Post-It Notes alike.

Jessie lives with her partner in an oceanfront cottage on the Eastern Shore of Nova Scotia, where they raise their children and tend to their land. *Project Body Love* is Jessie's first book.

Find out more about Jessie's work at

www.jessieharrold.com

Get in touch with Jessie via email at

jessie@jessieharrold.com

or on Instagram + Facebook @jessie.es.harrold

Spreading The Word

Independent publications rely on social proof and word-of-mouth to land in the hands of the people that can benefit from them the most. This book is no exception.

If you resonated with this book, please consider spreading the word. You can:

Leave a review on Amazon. This *dramatically* helps to increase this book's visibility. Head over to <u>amazon.com</u>, type "Project Body Love" in the search bar, and click on my book. Underneath the title, click on "customer reviews," and then click "write a review." THANK YOU!

Take a photo of this book as you're reading it and post it to Instagram. Use the hashtag #projectbodylove.

Write about *Project Body Love* on your blog, social media, or invite me to speak on your podcast.

Start a book club. Hold a women's circle. Have meaningful and honest conversations with the women in your life about how you feel about your body, and how you've been impacted by Diet Culture. Start with the questions on the next page and go from there. Also? I would love for you to reach out and tell me how it went, or share it on social media using the hashtag #projectbodylove.

Further Inquiry

It would be tempting to follow in Diet Culture's foot-steps and offer you a *"I can do it, you can do it, too"* twelve-step antidote to the complex and particular ways that you have struggled with living in your own body.

But, in many ways, your quest toward finding acceptance, respect and *maybe even love* for the skin you're in is unique to you.

You don't have to do this alone, though.

Here are a few of the questions that helped me plunge the depths of my relationship with my body. They can be answered privately, in your own journal, or in a book club or women's circle. My hope is that these will help you to uncover something new – a different perspective or a newfound sense of appreciation, perhaps, for your body.

What is the history of your relationship with your body? What pivotal moments in your past have shaped the way you feel about your body?

What are your values when it comes to your body (for example, your size and shape, ability and health). Where do these values come from?

How do you tend to your body's physical needs? What is your body calling to you for?

What is your purpose for your body?

Make a *fearless and searching inventory* of the things you know about your body.

If you could apologize to your body, what would you say?

What are you ready to forgive and let go of in order to deepen your relationship with your body?

What would be possible for you if you could reconnect with and reclaim your relationship with your body?

Deeper Still...

unEARTH is a three-month intensive program that supports women to reconnect with and reclaim who they are and what matters most to them, whether that's in their bodies, their careers, their relationships or their spirituality.

unEARTH uses the same methodology I used to reclaim my relationship with my body, intertwined with deep, experiential learning about the seven essential skills of the wise wild woman: self-tending, ritual, embodiment, earth connection, intuition, community, creativity and more.

During unEARTH, you'll engage in weekly virtual women's circles + lessons, have three intimate group coaching sessions, and be invited to change your life, one tiny experiment at a time.

To find out more, head to www.jessieharrold.com/unearth

Resources

Workbooks

The Body Sovereignty Workbook by Rachel Cole
Body Loving Homework by Mara Glatzel
The Intuitive Eating Workbook by Elise Resch and Evelyn Tribole

Podcasts, Video & Audio

The Fuck It Diet Podcast
Food Psych
Fearless Rebelle Radio
Real Talk Radio
Joyous Body by Clarissa Pinkola Estes
Dietland

Books

The Beauty Myth by Naomi Wolf
Face Value by Autumn Whitefield-Madrano
Intuitive Eating by Elise Resch and Evelyn Tribole
Curvy Yoga by Anna Guest-Jelley
Health at Every Size by Linda Bacon
Body Respect by Linda Bacon
Wild Feminine by Tami Lynn Kent
Love Warrior by Glennon Doyle Melton
Women Who Run With the Wolves by Clarissa Pinkola Estes
Dance of the Dissident Daughter by Sue Monk Kidd
Hunger by Roxane Gay
Self-Compassion by Kristen Neff

Landwhale by Jes Baker
You Have The Right to Remain Fat by Virgie Tovar
Shrill by Lindy West

Instagram

@unlikelyhikers
@nolatrees
@lvernon2000
@theashleygraham
@bodyposipanda
@the12ishstyle
@tallulah_moon
@allisonkimmey
@mynameisjessamyn
@torridfashion
@diannebondyyoga
@curvyyoga
@4thtribodies
@effyourbeautystandards
@themilitantbaker
@bodyimagemovement
@virgietovar
@summerinnanen
@chr1styharrison
@isabelfoxenduke
@maraglatzel
@ifd_bodies
@crushtheculture
@viviennemcm
@rachelwcole
@aidybryant

211

@mskelseymiller
@thefuckitdiet
@art.brat.comics
@fatgirlstraveling
@fatgirlshiking
@benourishedpdx
@adipositivity

Bibliography

Bacon L., Keim N.L., Van Loan M.D., et al. (2002). Evaluating a 'non-diet' wellness intervention for improvement of metabolic fitness, psychological well-being and eating and activity behaviors. *Int J Obes Relat Metab Disord. 26: 854-65.*

Bacon L., Stern J.S., Van Loan M.D., Keim N.L. (2005). Size acceptance and intuitive eating improve health for obese, female chronic dieters. *J Am Diet Assoc. 105: 929-36.*

Bombak, A. (2014). Obesity, Health at Every Size, and Public Health Policy. *American Journal of Public Health,* 104(2), 60-67.

Herman C.P., Polivy J., & Esses V.M. (1987). The illusion of counter-regulation. *Appetite,* 9, 161-169.

Van Dyke, N. & Drinkwater, E.J. (2014). Relationships between intuitive eating and health indicators: literature review. *Public Health Nutrition   17(8).*

Printed in Great Britain
by Amazon